CDT 2018

Dental Procedure Codes

ADA American Dental Association®
America's leading advocate for oral health

Table of Contents

Preface

Introduction

This reference manual, published by the ADA, contains the *Code on Dental Procedures and Nomenclature* (CDT Code) version that is effective for services provided on or after January 1, 2018 through December 31, 2018.

In August 2000 the CDT Code was designated by the federal government as the national terminology for reporting dental services on claims submitted to third-party payers, in accordance with authority granted by the Health Insurance Portability and Accountability Act of 1996 (HIPAA).

The ADA's Council on Dental Benefit Programs is responsible for maintaining the CDT Code in accordance with ADA Bylaws and policy, and applicable federal regulations. CDT Manual content is developed by the Council, while responsibility for CDT Manual printing, pricing and distribution of falls to the ADA's Department of Product Development and Sales.

- Should you have any recommendations for CDT Code **additions, revisions or deletions**, direct access to the process is via the portal established on the ADA web page *www.ADA.org/cdt*.

- For questions about dental procedure coding or claim submission call the ADA Member Service Center (members: toll free number on your membership card; non-members: 312.440.2500). Support is available from 8:30 a.m. to 5:00 p.m. Central Time, Monday through Friday.

- For general information about, or to pursue CDT Code **licensing,** please go to the ADA web page *www.ADA.org/en/publications/ada-catalog/cdt-products/licensing-for-commercial-users*. In addition to information about licensing this site contains the questionnaire that must be completed as the first step of the licensing process.

- For any questions regarding **pricing or purchasing** additional copies of the CDT Manual visit *www.adacatalog.org* or call 800-947-4746.

Preface

Categories of Service

The CDT Code is organized into twelve categories of service, each with its own series of five-digit alphanumeric codes:

Category of Service	Code Series
I. Diagnostic	D0100 – D0999
II. Preventive	D1000 – D1999
III. Restorative	D2000 – D2999
IV. Endodontics	D3000 – D3999
V. Periodontics	D4000 – D4999
VI. Prosthodontics, removable	D5000 – D5899
VII. Maxillofacial Prosthetics	D5900 – D5999
VIII. Implant Services	D6000 – D6199
IX. Prosthodontics, fixed	D6200 – D6999
X. Oral & Maxillofacial Surgery	D7000 – D7999
XI. Orthodontics	D8000 – D8999
XII. Adjunctive General Services	D9000 – D9999

These categories exist solely as a means to organize the CDT Code. As a result, some categories of service are divided into subcategories of related procedures. Many categories and subcategories have descriptors applicable to all procedure codes therein.

Dental procedure codes within a Category of Service, or a subcategory, are not always in numeric order. The reason is that existing numeric sequences often do not have unassigned codes available for CDT Code additions.

Components of a Dental Procedure Code Entry

Every procedure in the CDT Code must have the first two of the following three components:

1. **Procedure Code –** A five character alphanumeric code beginning with the letter "D" that identifies a specific dental procedure. A Procedure Code cannot be changed or abbreviated.

2. **Nomenclature –** The written title of a Procedure Code. Nomenclature may be abbreviated when printed on claim forms or other documents that are subject to space limitation. Any such abbreviation does not constitute a change to the Nomenclature.

3. **Descriptor –** A written narrative that further defines the nature and intended use of a single Procedure Code, or group of such codes. A Descriptor, when present, follows the applicable Procedure Code and its Nomenclature. Descriptors that apply to a series of Procedure Codes precede that series of codes.

Using the CDT Code

The following points should prove helpful when using the CDT Code for recording services provided on the patient record, and when reporting procedures on a paper or electronic claim submission.

1. The presence of a CDT Code does not mean that the procedure is:
   a. endorsed by any entity or is considered a standard of care
   b. covered or reimbursed by a dental benefits plan

2. General practitioners, specialists, and other individuals may report any of the listed CDT Codes as long as they are delivering procedures and services within the scope of their state law.

3. CDT Codes that require inclusion of a narrative description on the claim have the words "by report" in their nomenclature.

4. "Unspecified... procedure, by report" codes are used when, in the opinion of the dentist, there is no other CDT Code entry that accurately describes the services provided the patient.

Required Statement

If there is more than one code in this edition that consists of a procedure and a dentist submits a claim under one of these codes, the payor may process the claim under any of these codes that is consistent with the payor's reimbursement policy.

1

Code on Dental Procedures and Nomenclature

ADA American Dental Association®
America's leading advocate for oral health

Code on Dental Procedures and Nomenclature

The current version of the *Code on Dental Procedures and Nomenclature* (CDT Code) that follows is effective for the calendar year 2018. There are a number of changes from the prior version, which are identified by the following symbols:

- ● New procedure code
- ▲ Revision to a nomenclature or descriptor

Dental procedure codes that are no longer valid are not present. Chapter 2 contains the summary of all additions, revisions and deletions effective January 1, 2018.

As noted in the "Preface" the CDT Code is divided into twelve Categories of Service, and each category begins at the top of a right-hand page in this section of the manual.

Please note that when a code's nomenclature includes a "by report" notation, a narrative explaining the treatment provided must be included with the claim submission.

Classification of Materials

Names of dental materials are included in numerous procedure nomenclatures within several Categories of Service (e.g., Restorative; Prosthodontics, fixed). The following list of dental materials is included in the CDT Code **solely to aid selection** of a procedure code applicable to the service provided.

Classification of Metals (Source: ADA Council on Scientific Affairs online at: *www.ada.org/alloys*)

The noble metal classification system has been adopted as a more precise method of reporting various alloys used in dentistry. The alloys are defined on the basis of the percentage of metal content.

CLASSIFICATION	REQUIREMENT
High Noble Alloys	Noble Metal Content ≥ 60% (gold+ platinum group*) and gold ≥ 40%
Titanium and Titanium Alloys	Titanium ≥ 85%
Noble Alloys	Noble Metal Content ≥ 25% (gold + platinum group*)
Predominantly Base Alloys	Noble Metal Content < 25% (gold + platinum group*)

* metals of the platinum group are platinum, palladium, rhodium, iridium, osmium and ruthenium

Porcelain/ceramic
Refers to pressed, fired, polished or milled materials containing predominantly inorganic refractory compounds including porcelains, glasses, ceramics, and glass-ceramics.

Resin
Refers to any resin-based composite, including fiber or ceramic reinforced polymer compounds, and glass ionomers.

D0100-D0999   I. Diagnostic

Clinical Oral Evaluations

The codes in this section recognize the cognitive skills necessary for patient evaluation. The collection and recording of some data and components of the dental examination may be delegated; however, the evaluation, which includes diagnosis and treatment planning, is the responsibility of the dentist. As with all ADA procedure codes, there is no distinction made between the evaluations provided by general practitioners and specialists. Report additional diagnostic and/or definitive procedures separately.

D0120   periodic oral evaluation – established patient
An evaluation performed on a patient of record to determine any changes in the patient's dental and medical health status since a previous comprehensive or periodic evaluation. This includes an oral cancer evaluation and periodontal screening where indicated, and may require interpretation of information acquired through additional diagnostic procedures. Report additional diagnostic procedures separately.

D0140   limited oral evaluation – problem focused
An evaluation limited to a specific oral health problem or complaint. This may require interpretation of information acquired through additional diagnostic procedures. Report additional diagnostic procedures separately. Definitive procedures may be required on the same date as the evaluation.

Typically, patients receiving this type of evaluation present with a specific problem and/or dental emergencies, trauma, acute infections, etc.

D0145   oral evaluation for a patient under three years of age and counseling with primary caregiver
Diagnostic services performed for a child under the age of three, preferably within the first six months of the eruption of the first primary tooth, including recording the oral and physical health history, evaluation of caries susceptibility, development of an appropriate preventive oral health regimen and communication with and counseling of the child's parent, legal guardian and/or primary caregiver.

D0150 comprehensive oral evaluation – new or established patient
Used by a general dentist and/or a specialist when evaluating a patient comprehensively. This applies to new patients; established patients who have had a significant change in health conditions or other unusual circumstances, by report, or established patients who have been absent from active treatment for three or more years. It is a thorough evaluation and recording of the extraoral and intraoral hard and soft tissues. It may require interpretation of information acquired through additional diagnostic procedures. Additional diagnostic procedures should be reported separately.

This includes an evaluation for oral cancer where indicated, the evaluation and recording of the patient's dental and medical history and a general health assessment. It may include the evaluation and recording of dental caries, missing or unerupted teeth, restorations, existing prostheses, occlusal relationships, periodontal conditions (including periodontal screening and/or charting), hard and soft tissue anomalies, etc.

D0160 detailed and extensive oral evaluation – problem focused, by report
A detailed and extensive problem focused evaluation entails extensive diagnostic and cognitive modalities based on the findings of a comprehensive oral evaluation. Integration of more extensive diagnostic modalities to develop a treatment plan for a specific problem is required. The condition requiring this type of evaluation should be described and documented.

Examples of conditions requiring this type of evaluation may include dentofacial anomalies, complicated perio-prosthetic conditions, complex temporomandibular dysfunction, facial pain of unknown origin, conditions requiring multi-disciplinary consultation, etc.

D0170 re-evaluation – limited, problem focused (established patient; not post-operative visit)
Assessing the status of a previously existing condition. For example:

- a traumatic injury where no treatment was rendered but patient needs follow-up monitoring;

- evaluation for undiagnosed continuing pain;

- soft tissue lesion requiring follow-up evaluation.

● new procedure code   ▲ revision to a nomenclature or descriptor

D0171 **re-evaluation – post-operative office visit**

D0180 **comprehensive periodontal evaluation – new or established patient**
This procedure is indicated for patients showing signs or symptoms of periodontal disease and for patients with risk factors such as smoking or diabetes. It includes evaluation of periodontal conditions, probing and charting, evaluation and recording of the patient's dental and medical history and general health assessment. It may include the evaluation and recording of dental caries, missing or unerupted teeth, restorations, occlusal relationships and oral cancer evaluation.

Pre-diagnostic Services

D0190 **screening of a patient**
A screening, including state or federally mandated screenings, to determine an individual's need to be seen by a dentist for diagnosis.

D0191 **assessment of a patient**
A limited clinical inspection that is performed to identify possible signs of oral or systemic disease, malformation, or injury, and the potential need for referral for diagnosis and treatment.

Diagnostic Imaging

Should be taken only for clinical reasons as determined by the patient's dentist. Should be of diagnostic quality and properly identified and dated. Is a part of the patient's clinical record and the original images should be retained by the dentist. Originals should not be used to fulfill requests made by patients or third-parties for copies of records.

Image Capture with Interpretation

D0210 **intraoral – complete series of radiographic images**
A radiographic survey of the whole mouth, usually consisting of 14-22 periapical and posterior bitewing images intended to display the crowns and roots of all teeth, periapical areas and alveolar bone.

D0220 **intraoral – periapical first radiographic image**

D0230 intraoral – periapical each additional radiographic image

D0240 intraoral – occlusal radiographic image

D0250 extra-oral – 2D projection radiographic image created using a stationary radiation source, and detector
These images include, but are not limited to: Lateral Skull; Posterior-Anterior Skull; Submentovertex; Waters; Reverse Tomes; Oblique Mandibular Body; Lateral Ramus.

D0251 extra-oral posterior dental radiographic image
Image limited to exposure of complete posterior teeth in both dental arches. This is a unique image that is not derived from another image.

D0270 bitewing – single radiographic image

D0272 bitewings – two radiographic images

D0273 bitewings – three radiographic images

D0274 bitewings – four radiographic images

D0277 vertical bitewings – 7 to 8 radiographic images
This does not constitute a full mouth intraoral radiographic series.

D0310 sialography

D0320 temporomandibular joint arthrogram, including injection

D0321 other temporomandibular joint radiographic images, by report

D0322 tomographic survey

D0330 panoramic radiographic image

D0340 2D cephalometric radiographic image – acquisition, measurement and analysis
Image of the head made using a cephalostat to standardize anatomic positioning, and with reproducible x-ray beam geometry.

D0350 2D oral/facial photographic image obtained intra-orally or extra-orally

● new procedure code   ▲ revision to a nomenclature or descriptor

D0351 **3D photographic image**
This procedure is for dental or maxillofacial diagnostic purposes. Not applicable for a CAD-CAM procedure.

D0364 **cone beam CT capture and interpretation with limited field of view – less than one whole jaw**

D0365 **cone beam CT capture and interpretation with field of view of one full dental arch – mandible**

D0366 **cone beam CT capture and interpretation with field of view of one full dental arch – maxilla, with or without cranium**

D0367 **cone beam CT capture and interpretation with field of view of both jaws; with or without cranium**

D0368 **cone beam CT capture and interpretation for TMJ series including two or more exposures**

D0369 **maxillofacial MRI capture and interpretation**

D0370 **maxillofacial ultrasound capture and interpretation**

D0371 **sialoendoscopy capture and interpretation**

Image Capture Only

Capture by a Practitioner not associated with Interpretation and Report

D0380 **cone beam CT image capture with limited field of view – less than one whole jaw**

D0381 **cone beam CT image capture with field of view of one full dental arch – mandible**

D0382 **cone beam CT image capture with field of view of one full dental arch – maxilla, with or without cranium**

D0383 **cone beam CT image capture with field of view of both jaws, with or without cranium**

D0384 **cone beam CT image capture for TMJ series including two or more exposures**

D0385 **maxillofacial MRI image capture**

D0386 **maxillofacial ultrasound image capture**

Interpretation and Report Only
Interpretation and Report by a Practitioner not associated with Image Capture

D0391 **interpretation of diagnostic image by a practitioner not associated with capture of the image, including report**

Post Processing of Image or Image Sets

D0393 **treatment simulation using 3D image volume**
The use of 3D image volumes for simulation of treatment including, but not limited to, dental implant placement, orthognathic surgery and orthodontic tooth movement.

D0394 **digital subtraction of two or more images or image volumes of the same modality**
To demonstrate changes that have occurred over time.

D0395 **fusion of two or more 3D image volumes of one or more modalities**

Tests and Examinations

• **D0411** **HbA1c in-office point of service testing**

D0414 **laboratory processing of microbial specimen to include culture and sensitivity studies, preparation and transmission of written report**

D0415 **collection of microorganisms for culture and sensitivity**

D0416 **viral culture**
A diagnostic test to identify viral organisms, most often herpes virus.

D0417 **collection and preparation of saliva sample for laboratory diagnostic testing**

D0418 **analysis of saliva sample**
Chemical or biological analysis of saliva sample for diagnostic purposes.

D0422 **collection and preparation of genetic sample material for laboratory analysis and report**

D0423 **genetic test for susceptibility to diseases – specimen analysis**
Certified laboratory analysis to detect specific genetic variations associated with increased susceptibility for diseases.

D0425 **caries susceptibility tests**
Not to be used for carious dentin staining.

D0431 **adjunctive pre-diagnostic test that aids in detection of mucosal abnormalities including premalignant and malignant lesions, not to include cytology or biopsy procedures**

D0460 **pulp vitality tests**
Includes multiple teeth and contra lateral comparison(s), as indicated.

D0470 **diagnostic casts**
Also known as diagnostic models or study models.

D0600 **non-ionizing diagnostic procedure capable of quantifying, monitoring, and recording changes in structure of enamel, dentin, and cementum**

D0601 **caries risk assessment and documentation, with a finding of low risk**
Using recognized assessment tools.

D0602 **caries risk assessment and documentation, with a finding of moderate risk**
Using recognized assessment tools.

D0603 **caries risk assessment and documentation, with a finding of high risk**
Using recognized assessment tools.

Oral Pathology Laboratory

These procedures do not include collection of the tissue sample, which is documented separately.

D0472 **accession of tissue, gross examination, preparation and transmission of written report**
To be used in reporting architecturally intact tissue obtained by invasive means.

D0473 **accession of tissue, gross and microscopic examination, preparation and transmission of written report**
To be used in reporting architecturally intact tissue obtained by invasive means.

D0474 **accession of tissue, gross and microscopic examination, including assessment of surgical margins for presence of disease, preparation and transmission of written report**
To be used in reporting architecturally intact tissue obtained by invasive means.

D0480 **accession of exfoliative cytologic smears, microscopic examination, preparation and transmission of written report**
To be used in reporting disaggregated, non-transepithelial cell cytology sample via mild scraping of the oral mucosa.

D0486 **laboratory accession of transepithelial cytologic sample, microscopic examination, preparation and transmission of written report**
Analysis, and written report of findings, of cytological sample of disaggregated transepithelial cells.

D0475 **decalcification procedure**
Procedure in which hard tissue is processed in order to allow sectioning and subsequent microscopic examination.

D0476 **special stains for microorganisms**
Procedure in which additional stains are applied to biopsy or surgical specimen in order to identify microorganisms.

● new procedure code   ▲ revision to a nomenclature or descriptor

D0477 **special stains, not for microorganisms**
Procedure in which additional stains are applied to a biopsy or surgical specimen in order to identify such things as melanin, mucin, iron, glycogen, etc.

D0478 **immunohistochemical stains**
A procedure in which specific antibody based reagents are applied to tissue samples in order to facilitate diagnosis.

D0479 **tissue in-situ hybridization, including interpretation**
A procedure which allows for the identification of nucleic acids, DNA and RNA, in the tissue sample in order to aid in the diagnosis of microorganisms and tumors.

D0481 **electron microscopy**

D0482 **direct immunofluorescence**
A technique used to identify immunoreactants which are localized to the patient's skin or mucous membranes.

D0483 **indirect immunofluorescence**
A technique used to identify circulating immunoreactants.

D0484 **consultation on slides prepared elsewhere**
A service provided in which microscopic slides of a biopsy specimen prepared at another laboratory are evaluated to aid in the diagnosis of a difficult case or to offer a consultative opinion at the patient's request. The findings are delivered by written report.

D0485 **consultation, including preparation of slides from biopsy material supplied by referring source**
A service that requires the consulting pathologist to prepare the slides as well as render a written report. The slides are evaluated to aid in the diagnosis of a difficult case or to offer a consultative opinion at the patient's request.

D0502 **other oral pathology procedures, by report**

D0999 **unspecified diagnostic procedure, by report**
Used for procedure that is not adequately described by a code. Describe procedure.

D1000–D1999 II. Preventive

Dental Prophylaxis

D1110 **prophylaxis – adult**
Removal of plaque, calculus and stains from the tooth structures in the permanent and transitional dentition. It is intended to control local irritational factors.

D1120 **prophylaxis – child**
Removal of plaque, calculus and stains from the tooth structures in the primary and transitional dentition. It is intended to control local irritational factors.

Topical Fluoride Treatment (Office Procedure)

Prescription strength fluoride product designed solely for use in the dental office, delivered to the dentition under the direct supervision of a dental professional. Fluoride must be applied separately from prophylaxis paste.

D1206 **topical application of fluoride varnish**

D1208 **topical application of fluoride – excluding varnish**

Other Preventive Services

D1310 **nutritional counseling for control of dental disease**
Counseling on food selection and dietary habits as a part of treatment and control of periodontal disease and caries.

D1320 **tobacco counseling for the control and prevention of oral disease**
Tobacco prevention and cessation services reduce patient risks of developing tobacco-related oral diseases and conditions and improves prognosis for certain dental therapies.

D1330 **oral hygiene instructions**
This may include instructions for home care. Examples include tooth brushing technique, flossing, and use of special oral hygiene aids.

D1351 **sealant – per tooth**
Mechanically and/or chemically prepared enamel surface sealed to prevent decay.

D1353 **sealant repair – per tooth**

D1352 **preventive resin restoration in a moderate to high caries risk patient – permanent tooth**
Conservative restoration of an active cavitated lesion in a pit or fissure that does not extend into dentin; includes placement of a sealant in any radiating non-carious fissures or pits.

▲ **D1354** **interim caries arresting medicament application – per tooth**
Conservative treatment of an active, non-symptomatic carious lesion by topical application of a caries arresting or inhibiting medicament and without mechanical removal of sound tooth structure.

Space Maintenance (Passive Appliances)

Passive appliances are designed to prevent tooth movement.

D1510 **space maintainer – fixed, unilateral**
Excludes a distal shoe space maintainer.

D1515 **space maintainer – fixed - bilateral**

D1520 **space maintainer – removable – unilateral**

D1525 **space maintainer – removable – bilateral**

D1550 **re-cement or re-bond space maintainer**

▲ **D1555** **removal of fixed space maintainer**
Procedure performed by dentist or practice that did not originally place the appliance.

● new procedure code   ▲ revision to a nomenclature or descriptor

Space Maintainers

D1575 **distal shoe space maintainer – fixed – unilateral**
Fabrication and delivery of fixed appliance extending subgingivally
and distally to guide the eruption of the first permanent molar.
Does not include ongoing follow-up or adjustments, or replacement
appliances, once the tooth has erupted.

D1999 **unspecified preventive procedure, by report**
Used for procedure that is not adequately described by another
CDT Code. Describe procedure.

D2000-D2999 III. Restorative

Local anesthesia is usually considered to be part of Restorative procedures.

Explanation of Restorations

Location	Number of Surfaces	Characteristics
Anterior	1	Placed on one of the following five surface classifications – Mesial, Distal, Incisal, Lingual, or Facial (or Labial).
	2	Placed, without interruption, on two of the five surface classifications – e.g., Mesial-Lingual.
	3	Placed, without interruption, on three of the five surface classifications – e.g., Lingual-Mesial-Facial (or Labial).
	4 or more	Placed, without interruption, on four or more of the five surface classifications – e.g., Mesial-Incisal-Lingual-Facial (or Labial).
Posterior	1	Placed on one of the following five surface classifications – Mesial, Distal, Occlusal, Lingual, or Buccal.
	2	Placed, without interruption, on two of the five surface classifications – e.g., Mesial-Occlusal.
	3	Placed, without interruption, on three of the five surface classifications – e.g., Lingual-Occlusal-Distal.
	4 or more	Placed, without interruption, on four or more of the five surface classifications – e.g., Mesial-Occlusal-Lingual-Distal.

Note: Tooth surfaces are reported on the HIPAA standard electronic dental transaction and the ADA Dental Claim Form using the letters in the following table.

Surface	Code
Buccal	B
Distal	D
Facial (or Labial)	F
Incisal	I
Lingual	L
Mesial	M
Occlusal	O

Amalgam Restorations (Including Polishing)

Tooth preparation, all adhesives (including amalgam bonding agents), liners and bases are included as part of the restoration. If pins are used, they should be reported separately (see D2951).

D2140 **amalgam – one surface, primary or permanent**

D2150 **amalgam – two surfaces, primary or permanent**

D2160 **amalgam – three surfaces, primary or permanent**

D2161 **amalgam – four or more surfaces, primary or permanent**

Resin-Based Composite Restorations – Direct

Resin-based composite refers to a broad category of materials including but not limited to composites. May include bonded composite, light-cured composite, etc. Tooth preparation, acid etching, adhesives (including resin bonding agents), liners and bases and curing are included as part of the restoration. Glass ionomers, when used as restorations, should be reported with these codes. If pins are used, they should be reported separately (see D2951).

D2330 **resin-based composite – one surface, anterior**

D2331 **resin-based composite – two surfaces, anterior**

D2332 **resin-based composite – three surfaces, anterior**

D2335 **resin-based composite – four or more surfaces or involving incisal angle (anterior)**
Incisal angle to be defined as one of the angles formed by the junction of the incisal and the mesial or distal surface of an anterior tooth.

D2390 **resin-based composite crown, anterior**
Full resin-based composite coverage of tooth.

D2391 **resin-based composite – one surface, posterior**
Used to restore a carious lesion into the dentin or a deeply eroded area into the dentin. Not a preventive procedure.

D2392 **resin-based composite – two surfaces, posterior**

D2393 **resin-based composite – three surfaces, posterior**

D2394 **resin-based composite – four or more surfaces, posterior**

Gold Foil Restorations

D2410 **gold foil – one surface**

D2420 **gold foil – two surfaces**

D2430 **gold foil – three surfaces**

Inlay/Onlay Restorations

Inlay: An intra-coronal dental restoration, made outside the oral cavity to conform to the prepared cavity, which does not restore any cusp tips.

Onlay: A dental restoration made outside the oral cavity that covers one or more cusp tips and adjoining occlusal surfaces, but not the entire external surface.

D2510 **inlay – metallic – one surface**

D2520 **inlay – metallic – two surfaces**

D2530 **inlay – metallic – three or more surfaces**

D2542 **onlay – metallic – two surfaces**

D2543 **onlay – metallic – three surfaces**

D2544 **onlay – metallic – four or more surfaces**

Porcelain/ceramic inlays/onlays include all indirect ceramic and porcelain type inlays/onlays.

D2610 **inlay – porcelain/ceramic – one surface**

D2620 **inlay – porcelain/ceramic – two surfaces**

D2630 **inlay – porcelain/ceramic – three or more surfaces**

D2642 **onlay – porcelain/ceramic – two surfaces**

D2643 onlay – porcelain/ceramic – three surfaces

D2644 onlay – porcelain/ceramic – four or more surfaces

Resin-based composite inlays/onlays must utilize
indirect technique.

D2650 inlay – resin-based composite – one surface

D2651 inlay – resin-based composite – two surfaces

D2652 inlay – resin-based composite – three or more surfaces

D2662 onlay – resin-based composite – two surfaces

D2663 onlay – resin-based composite – three surfaces

D2664 onlay – resin-based composite – four or more surfaces

Crowns – Single Restorations Only

D2710 crown – resin-based composite (indirect)

D2712 crown – ¾ resin-based composite (indirect)
This procedure does not include facial veneers.

D2720 crown – resin with high noble metal

D2721 crown – resin with predominantly base metal

D2722 crown – resin with noble metal

▲ **D2740** crown – porcelain/ceramic

D2750 crown – porcelain fused to high noble metal

D2751 crown – porcelain fused to predominantly base metal

D2752 crown – porcelain fused to noble metal

D2780 crown – ¾ cast high noble metal

D2781 crown – ¾ cast predominantly base metal

D2782 crown – ¾ cast noble metal

D2783 crown – ¾ porcelain/ceramic
This procedure does not include facial veneers.

D2790 crown – full cast high noble metal

D2791 crown – full cast predominantly base metal

D2792 crown – full cast noble metal

D2794 crown – titanium

D2799 provisional crown– further treatment or completion of diagnosis necessary prior to final impression
Not to be used as a temporary crown for a routine prosthetic restoration.

Other Restorative Services

D2990 resin infiltration of incipient smooth surface lesions
Placement of an infiltrating resin restoration for strengthening, stabilizing and/or limiting the progression of the lesion.

D2910 re-cement or re-bond inlay, onlay, veneer or partial coverage restoration

D2915 re-cement or re-bond indirectly fabricated or prefabricated post and core

D2920 re-cement or re-bond crown

D2921 reattachment of tooth fragment, incisal edge or cusp

D2929 prefabricated porcelain/ceramic crown – primary tooth

D2930 prefabricated stainless steel crown – primary tooth

D2931 prefabricated stainless steel crown – permanent tooth

D2932 prefabricated resin crown

D2933 **prefabricated stainless steel crown with resin window**
Open-face stainless steel crown with aesthetic resin facing or veneer.

D2934 **prefabricated esthetic coated stainless steel crown – primary tooth**
Stainless steel primary crown with exterior esthetic coating.

D2940 **protective restoration**
Direct placement of a restorative material to protect tooth and/or tissue form. This procedure may be used to relieve pain, promote healing, or prevent further deterioration. Not to be used for endodontic access closure, or as a base or liner under restoration.

D2941 **interim therapeutic restoration – primary dentition**
Placement of an adhesive restorative material following caries debridement by hand or other method for the management of early childhood caries. Not considered a definitive restoration.

D2949 **restorative foundation for an indirect restoration**
Placement of restorative material to yield a more ideal form, including elimination of undercuts.

D2950 **core buildup, including any pins when required**
Refers to building up of coronal structure when there is insufficient retention for a separate extracoronal restorative procedure. A core buildup is not a filler to eliminate any undercut, box form, or concave irregularity in a preparation.

D2951 **pin retention – per tooth, in addition to restoration**

D2952 **post and core in addition to crown, indirectly fabricated**
Post and core are custom fabricated as a single unit.

D2953 **each additional indirectly fabricated post – same tooth**
To be used with D2952.

D2954 **prefabricated post and core in addition to crown**
Core is built around a prefabricated post. This procedure includes the core material.

D2957 each additional prefabricated post – same tooth
To be used with D2954.

D2955 post removal

D2960 labial veneer (resin laminate) – chairside
Refers to labial/facial direct resin bonded veneers.

D2961 labial veneer (resin laminate) – laboratory
Refers to labial/facial indirect resin bonded veneers.

D2962 labial veneer (porcelain laminate) – laboratory
Refers also to facial veneers that extend interproximally and/or cover the incisal edge. Porcelain/ceramic veneers presently include all ceramic and porcelain veneers.

D2971 additional procedures to construct new crown under existing partial denture framework
To be reported in addition to a crown code.

D2975 coping
A thin covering of the coronal portion of a tooth, usually devoid of anatomic contour, that can be used as a definitive restoration.

D2980 crown repair necessitated by restorative material failure

D2981 inlay repair necessitated by restorative material failure

D2982 onlay repair necessitated by restorative material failure

D2983 veneer repair necessitated by restorative material failure

D2999 unspecified restorative procedure, by report
Use for procedure that is not adequately described by a code. Describe procedure.

D3000-D3999   IV. Endodontics

Local anesthesia is usually considered to be part of Endodontic procedures.

Pulp Capping

D3110   pulp cap – direct (excluding final restoration)
Procedure in which the exposed pulp is covered with a dressing or cement that protects the pulp and promotes healing and repair.

D3120   pulp cap – indirect (excluding final restoration)
Procedure in which the nearly exposed pulp is covered with a protective dressing to protect the pulp from additional injury and to promote healing and repair via formation of secondary dentin. This code is not to be used for bases and liners when all caries has been removed.

Pulpotomy

D3220   therapeutic pulpotomy (excluding final restoration) – removal of pulp coronal to the dentinocemental junction and application of medicament
Pulpotomy is the surgical removal of a portion of the pulp with the aim of maintaining the vitality of the remaining portion by means of an adequate dressing.

– To be performed on primary or permanent teeth.

– This is not to be construed as the first stage of root canal therapy.

– Not to be used for apexogenesis.

D3221   pulpal debridement, primary and permanent teeth
Pulpal debridement for the relief of acute pain prior to conventional root canal therapy. This procedure is not to be used when endodontic treatment is completed on the same day.

D3222 partial pulpotomy for apexogenesis – permanent tooth with incomplete root development
Removal of a portion of the pulp and application of a medicament with the aim of maintaining the vitality of the remaining portion to encourage continued physiological development and formation of the root. This procedure is not to be construed as the first stage of root canal therapy.

Endodontic Therapy on Primary Teeth

Endodontic therapy on primary teeth with succedaneous teeth and placement of resorbable filling. This includes pulpectomy, cleaning, and filling of canals with resorbable material.

D3230 pulpal therapy (resorbable filling) – anterior, primary tooth (excluding final restoration)
Primary incisors and cuspids.

D3240 pulpal therapy (resorbable filling) – posterior, primary tooth (excluding final restoration)
Primary first and second molars.

Endodontic Therapy (Including Treatment Plan, Clinical Procedures and Follow-Up Care)

Includes primary teeth without succedaneous teeth and permanent teeth. Complete root canal therapy; pulpectomy is part of root canal therapy.

Includes all appointments necessary to complete treatment; also includes intra-operative radiographs. Does not include diagnostic evaluation and necessary radiographs/diagnostic images.

D3310 endodontic therapy, anterior tooth (excluding final restoration)

▲ **D3320 endodontic therapy, premolar tooth (excluding final restoration)**

▲ **D3330** **endodontic therapy, molar tooth (excluding final restoration)**

D3331 **treatment of root canal obstruction; non-surgical access**
In lieu of surgery, the formation of a pathway to achieve an apical seal without surgical intervention because of a non-negotiable root canal blocked by foreign bodies, including but not limited to separated instruments, broken posts or calcification of 50% or more of the length of the tooth root.

D3332 **incomplete endodontic therapy; inoperable, unrestorable or fractured tooth**
Considerable time is necessary to determine diagnosis and/or provide initial treatment before the fracture makes the tooth unretainable.

D3333 **internal root repair of perforation defects**
Non-surgical seal of perforation caused by resorption and/or decay but not iatrogenic by provider filing claim.

Endodontic Retreatment

D3346 **retreatment of previous root canal therapy – anterior**

▲ **D3347** **retreatment of previous root canal therapy – premolar**

D3348 **retreatment of previous root canal therapy – molar**

Apexification/Recalcification

D3351 **apexification/recalcification – initial visit (apical closure/ calcific repair of perforations, root resorption, etc.)**
Includes opening tooth, preparation of canal spaces, first placement of medication and necessary radiographs. (This procedure may include first phase of complete root canal therapy.)

D3352 **apexification/recalcification – interim medication replacement**
For visits in which the intra-canal medication is replaced with new medication. Includes any necessary radiographs.

D3353 apexification/recalcification – final visit (includes completed root canal therapy – apical closure/calcific repair of perforations, root resorption, etc.)
Includes removal of intra-canal medication and procedures necessary to place final root canal filling material including necessary radiographs. (This procedure includes last phase of complete root canal therapy.)

Pulpal Regeneration

D3355 pulpal regeneration – initial visit
Includes opening tooth, preparation of canal spaces, placement of medication.

D3356 pulpal regeneration – interim medication replacement

D3357 pulpal regeneration – completion of treatment
Does not include final restoration.

Apicoectomy/Periradicular Services

Periradicular surgery is a term used to describe surgery to the root surface (e.g., apicoectomy), repair of a root perforation or resorptive defect, exploratory curettage to look for root fractures, removal of extruded filling materials or instruments, removal of broken root fragments, sealing of accessory canals, etc. This does not include retrograde filling material placement.

D3410 apicoectomy – anterior
For surgery on root of anterior tooth. Does not include placement of retrograde filling material.

▲ **D3421 apicoectomy – premolar (first root)**
For surgery on one root of a premolar. Does not include placement of retrograde filling material. If more than one root is treated, see D3426.

D3425 apicoectomy – molar (first root)
For surgery on one root of a molar tooth. Does not include placement of retrograde filling material. If more than one root is treated, see D3426.

▲ **D3426   apicoectomy (each additional root)**
Typically used for premolar and molar surgeries when more than one root is treated during the same procedure. This does not include retrograde filling material placement.

D3427   periradicular surgery without apicoectomy

D3428   bone graft in conjunction with periradicular surgery – per tooth, single site
Includes non-autogenous graft material.

D3429   bone graft in conjunction with periradicular surgery – each additional contiguous tooth in the same surgical site
Includes non-autogenous graft material.

D3430   retrograde filling – per root
For placement of retrograde filling material during periradicular surgery procedures. If more than one filling is placed in one root report as D3999 and describe.

D3431   biologic materials to aid in soft and osseous tissue regeneration in conjunction with periradicular surgery

D3432   guided tissue regeneration, resorbable barrier, per site, in conjunction with periradicular surgery

D3450   root amputation – per root
Root resection of a multi-rooted tooth while leaving the crown. If the crown is sectioned, see D3920.

D3460   endodontic endosseous implant
Placement of implant material, which extends from a pulpal space into the bone beyond the end of the root.

D3470   intentional re-implantation (including necessary splinting)
For the intentional removal, inspection and treatment of the root and replacement of a tooth into its own socket. This does not include necessary retrograde filling material placement.

Other Endodontic Procedures

D3910 surgical procedure for isolation of tooth with rubber dam

D3920 hemisection (including any root removal), not including root canal therapy
Includes separation of a multi-rooted tooth into separate sections containing the root and the overlying portion of the crown. It may also include the removal of one or more of those sections.

D3950 canal preparation and fitting of preformed dowel or post
Should not be reported in conjunction with D2952, D2953, D2954 or D2957 by the same practitioner.

D3999 unspecified endodontic procedure, by report
Used for procedure that is not adequately described by a code. Describe procedure.

D4000-D4999 V. Periodontics

Local anesthesia is usually considered to be part of Periodontal procedures.

Surgical Services (Including Usual Postoperative Care)

Site: A term used to describe a single area, position, or locus. The word "site" is frequently used to indicate an area of soft tissue recession on a single tooth or an osseous defect adjacent to a single tooth; also used to indicate soft tissue defects and/or osseous defects in edentulous tooth positions.

– If two contiguous teeth have areas of soft tissue recession, each area of recession is a single site.

– If two contiguous teeth have adjacent but separate osseous defects, each defect is a single site.

– If two contiguous teeth have a communicating interproximal osseous defect, it should be considered a single site.

– All non-communicating osseous defects are single sites.

– All edentulous non-contiguous tooth positions are single sites.

– Depending on the dimensions of the defect, up to two contiguous edentulous tooth positions may be considered a single site.

Tooth Bounded Space: A space created by one or more missing teeth that has a tooth on each side.

D4210 **gingivectomy or gingivoplasty – four or more contiguous teeth or tooth bounded spaces per quadrant**
It is performed to eliminate suprabony pockets or to restore normal architecture when gingival enlargements or asymmetrical or unaesthetic topography is evident with normal bony configuration.

D4211 **gingivectomy or gingivoplasty – one to three contiguous teeth or tooth bounded spaces per quadrant**
It is performed to eliminate suprabony pockets or to restore normal architecture when gingival enlargements or asymmetrical or unaesthetic topography is evident with normal bony configuration.

D4212 **gingivectomy or gingivoplasty to allow access for restorative procedure, per tooth**

▲ **D4230** **anatomical crown exposure – four or more contiguous teeth or bounded tooth spaces per quadrant**
This procedure is utilized in an otherwise periodontally healthy area to remove enlarged gingival tissue and supporting bone (ostectomy) to provide an anatomically correct gingival relationship.

▲ **D4231** **anatomical crown exposure – one to three teeth or bounded tooth spaces per quadrant**
This procedure is utilized in an otherwise periodontally healthy area to remove enlarged gingival tissue and supporting bone (ostectomy) to provide an anatomically correct gingival relationship.

D4240 **gingival flap procedure, including root planing – four or more contiguous teeth or tooth bounded spaces per quadrant**
A soft tissue flap is reflected or resected to allow debridement of the root surface and the removal of granulation tissue. Osseous recontouring is not accomplished in conjunction with this procedure. May include open flap curettage, reverse bevel flap surgery, modified Kirkland flap procedure, and modified Widman surgery. This procedure is performed in the presence of moderate to deep probing depths, loss of attachment, need to maintain esthetics, need for increased access to the root surface and alveolar bone, or to determine the presence of a cracked tooth, fractured root, or external root resorption. Other procedures may be required concurrent to D4240 and should be reported separately using their own unique codes.

D4241 **gingival flap procedure, including root planing – one to three contiguous teeth or tooth bounded spaces per quadrant**
A soft tissue flap is reflected or resected to allow debridement of the root surface and the removal of granulation tissue. Osseous recontouring is not accomplished in conjunction with this procedure. May include open flap curettage, reverse bevel flap surgery, modified Kirkland flap procedure, and modified Widman surgery. This procedure is performed in the presence of moderate to deep probing depths, loss of attachment, need to maintain esthetics, need for increased access to the root surface and alveolar bone, or to determine the presence of a cracked tooth, fractured root, or external root resorption. Other procedures may be required concurrent to D4241 and should be reported separately using their own unique codes.

D4245 **apically positioned flap**
Procedure is used to preserve keratinized gingiva in conjunction with osseous resection and second stage implant procedure. Procedure may also be used to preserve keratinized/attached gingiva during surgical exposure of labially impacted teeth, and may be used during treatment of peri-implantitis.

D4249 **clinical crown lengthening – hard tissue**
This procedure is employed to allow a restorative procedure on a tooth with little or no tooth structure exposed to the oral cavity. Crown lengthening requires reflection of a full thickness flap and removal of bone, altering the crown to root ratio. It is performed in a healthy periodontal environment, as opposed to osseous surgery, which is performed in the presence of periodontal disease.

D4260 **osseous surgery (including elevation of a full thickness flap and closure) – four or more contiguous teeth or tooth bounded spaces per quadrant**
This procedure modifies the bony support of the teeth by reshaping the alveolar process to achieve a more physiologic form during the surgical procedure. This must include the removal of supporting bone (ostectomy) and/or non-supporting bone (osteoplasty). Other procedures may be required concurrent to D4260 and should be reported using their own unique codes.

D4261 **osseous surgery (including elevation of a full thickness flap and closure) – one to three contiguous teeth or tooth bounded spaces per quadrant**
This procedure modifies the bony support of the teeth by reshaping the alveolar process to achieve a more physiologic form during the surgical procedure. This must include the removal of supporting bone (ostectomy) and/or non-supporting bone (osteoplasty). Other procedures may be required concurrent to D4261 and should be reported using their own unique codes.

D4263 **bone replacement graft – retained natural tooth – first site in quadrant**

This procedure involves the use of grafts to stimulate periodontal regeneration when the disease process has led to a deformity of the bone. This procedure does not include flap entry and closure, wound debridement, osseous contouring, or the placement of biologic materials to aid in osseous tissue regeneration or barrier membranes. Other separate procedures delivered concurrently are documented with their own codes. Not to be reported for an edentulous space or an extraction site.

D4264 **bone replacement graft – retained natural tooth – each additional site in quadrant**

This procedure involves the use of grafts to stimulate periodontal regeneration when the disease process has led to a deformity of the bone. This procedure does not include flap entry and closure, wound debridement, osseous contouring, or the placement of biologic materials to aid in osseous tissue regeneration or barrier membranes. This procedure is performed concurrently with one or more bone replacement grafts to document the number of sites involved. Not to be reported for an edentulous space or an extraction site.

D4265 **biologic materials to aid in soft and osseous tissue regeneration**

Biologic materials may be used alone or with other regenerative substrates such as bone and barrier membranes, depending upon their formulation and the presentation of the periodontal defect. This procedure does not include surgical entry and closure, wound debridement, osseous contouring, or the placement of graft materials and/or barrier membranes. Other separate procedures may be required concurrent to D4265 and should be reported using their own unique codes.

D4266 **guided tissue regeneration – resorbable barrier, per site**

This procedure does not include flap entry and closure, or, when indicated, wound debridement, osseous contouring, bone replacement grafts, and placement of biologic materials to aid in osseous regeneration. This procedure can be used for periodontal and peri-implant defects.

● new procedure code   ▲ revision to a nomenclature or descriptor

D4267 **guided tissue regeneration – non-resorbable barrier, per site (includes membrane removal)**
This procedure does not include flap entry and closure, or, when indicated, wound debridement, osseous contouring, bone replacement grafts, and placement of biologic materials to aid in osseous regeneration. This procedure can be used for periodontal and peri-implant defects.

D4268 **surgical revision procedure, per tooth**
This procedure is to refine the results of a previously provided surgical procedure. This may require a surgical procedure to modify the irregular contours of hard or soft tissue. A mucoperiosteal flap may be elevated to allow access to reshape alveolar bone. The flaps are replaced or repositioned and sutured.

D4270 **pedicle soft tissue graft procedure**
A pedicle flap of gingiva can be raised from an edentulous ridge, adjacent teeth, or from the existing gingiva on the tooth and moved laterally or coronally to replace alveolar mucosa as marginal tissue. The procedure can be used to cover an exposed root or to eliminate a gingival defect if the root is not too prominent in the arch.

D4273 **autogenous connective tissue graft procedure (including donor and recipient surgical sites) first tooth, implant or edentulous tooth position in graft**
There are two surgical sites. The recipient site utilizes a split thickness incision, retaining the overlapping flap of gingiva and/or mucosa. The connective tissue is dissected from a separate donor site leaving an epithelialized flap for closure.

D4283 **autogenous connective tissue graft procedure (including donor and recipient surgical sites) – each additional contiguous tooth, implant or edentulous tooth position in same graft site**
Used in conjunction with D4273.

D4275 **non-autogenous connective tissue graft (including recipient site and donor material) first tooth, implant, or edentulous tooth position in graft**
There is only a recipient surgical site utilizing split thickness incision, retaining the overlaying flap of gingiva and/or mucosa. A donor surgical site is not present.

D4285 **non-autogenous connective tissue graft procedure (including recipient surgical site and donor material) – each additional contiguous tooth, implant or edentulous tooth position in same graft site**
Used in conjunction with D4275.

D4274 **mesial/distal wedge procedure, single tooth (when not performed in conjunction with surgical procedures in the same anatomical area)**
This procedure is performed in an edentulous area adjacent to a tooth, allowing removal of a tissue wedge to gain access for debridement, permit close flap adaptation, and reduce pocket depths.

D4276 **combined connective tissue and double pedicle graft, per tooth**
Advanced gingival recession often cannot be corrected with a single procedure. Combined tissue grafting procedures are needed to achieve the desired outcome.

D4277 **free soft tissue graft procedure (including recipient and donor surgical sites) first tooth, implant, or edentulous tooth position in graft**

D4278 **free soft tissue graft procedure (including recipient and donor surgical sites) each additional contiguous tooth, implant, or edentulous tooth position in same graft site**
Used in conjunction with D4277.

Non-Surgical Periodontal Service

D4320 **provisional splinting – intracoronal**
This is an interim stabilization of mobile teeth. A variety of methods and appliances may be employed for this purpose. Identify the teeth involved.

D4321 **provisional splinting – extracoronal**
This is an interim stabilization of mobile teeth. A variety of methods and appliances may be employed for this purpose. Identify the teeth involved.

● new procedure code ▲ revision to a nomenclature or descriptor

D4341 **periodontal scaling and root planing – four or more teeth per quadrant**
This procedure involves instrumentation of the crown and root surfaces of the teeth to remove plaque and calculus from these surfaces. It is indicated for patients with periodontal disease and is therapeutic, not prophylactic, in nature. Root planing is the definitive procedure designed for the removal of cementum and dentin that is rough, and/or permeated by calculus or contaminated with toxins or microorganisms. Some soft tissue removal occurs. This procedure may be used as a definitive treatment in some stages of periodontal disease and/or as a part of pre-surgical procedures in others.

D4342 **periodontal scaling and root planing – one to three teeth per quadrant**
This procedure involves instrumentation of the crown and root surfaces of the teeth to remove plaque and calculus from these surfaces. It is indicated for patients with periodontal disease and is therapeutic, not prophylactic, in nature. Root planing is the definitive procedure designed for the removal of cementum and dentin that is rough, and/or permeated by calculus or contaminated with toxins or microorganisms. Some soft tissue removal occurs. This procedure may be used as a definitive treatment in some stages of periodontal disease and/or as a part of pre-surgical procedures in others.

D4346 **scaling in presence of generalized moderate or severe gingival inflammation – full mouth, after oral evaluation**
The removal of plaque, calculus and stains from supra- and sub-gingival tooth surfaces when there is generalized moderate or severe gingival inflammation in the absence of periodontitis. It is indicated for patients who have swollen, inflamed gingiva, generalized suprabony pockets, and moderate to severe bleeding on probing. Should not be reported in conjunction with prophylaxis, scaling and root planing, or debridement procedures.

▲ **D4355** **full mouth debridement to enable a comprehensive evaluation and diagnosis on a subsequent visit**
Full mouth debridement involves the preliminary removal of plaque and calculus that interferes with the ability of the dentist to perform a comprehensive oral evaluation. Not to be completed on the same day as D0150, D0160, or D0180.

D4381 **localized delivery of antimicrobial agents via a controlled release vehicle into diseased crevicular tissue, per tooth**
FDA approved subgingival delivery devices containing antimicrobial medication(s) are inserted into periodontal pockets to suppress the pathogenic microbiota. These devices slowly release the pharmacological agents so they can remain at the intended site of action in a therapeutic concentration for a sufficient length of time.

Other Periodontal Services

D4910 **periodontal maintenance**
This procedure is instituted following periodontal therapy and continues at varying intervals, determined by the clinical evaluation of the dentist, for the life of the dentition or any implant replacements. It includes removal of the bacterial plaque and calculus from supragingival and subgingival regions, site specific scaling and root planing where indicated, and polishing the teeth. If new or recurring periodontal disease appears, additional diagnostic and treatment procedures must be considered.

D4920 **unscheduled dressing change (by someone other than treating dentist or their staff)**

D4921 **gingival irrigation – per quadrant**
Irrigation of gingival pockets with medicinal agent. Not to be used to report use of mouth rinses or non-invasive chemical debridement.

D4999 **unspecified periodontal procedure, by report**
Use for procedure that is not adequately described by a code. Describe procedure.

● new procedure code   ▲ revision to a nomenclature or descriptor

D5000-D5899 VI. Prosthodontics (removable)

Local anesthesia is usually considered to be part of Removable Prosthodontic procedures.

Complete Dentures (Including Routine Post-Delivery Care)

D5110   **complete denture – maxillary**

D5120   **complete denture – mandibular**

D5130   **immediate denture – maxillary**
Includes limited follow-up care only; does not include future rebasing/relining procedure(s).

D5140   **immediate denture – mandibular**
Includes limited follow-up care only; does not include future rebasing/relining procedure(s).

Partial Dentures (Including Routine Post-Delivery Care)

D5211   **maxillary partial denture – resin base (including any conventional clasps, rests and teeth)**
Includes acrylic resin base denture with resin or wrought wire clasps.

D5212   **mandibular partial denture – resin base (including any conventional clasps, rests and teeth)**
Includes acrylic resin base denture with resin or wrought wire clasps.

D5213   **maxillary partial denture – cast metal framework with resin denture bases (including any conventional clasps, rests and teeth)**

D5214   **mandibular partial denture – cast metal framework with resin denture bases (including any conventional clasps, rests and teeth)**

D5221   **immediate maxillary partial denture – resin base (including any conventional clasps, rests and teeth)**
Includes limited follow-up care only; does not include future rebasing/relining procedure(s).

D5222   **immediate mandibular partial denture – resin base (including any conventional clasps, rests and teeth)**
Includes limited follow-up care only; does not include future rebasing/relining procedure(s).

D5223   **immediate maxillary partial denture – cast metal framework with resin denture bases (including any conventional clasps, rests and teeth**
Includes limited follow-up care only; does not include future rebasing/relining procedure(s).

D5224   **immediate mandibular partial denture – cast metal framework with resin denture bases (including any conventional clasps, rests and teeth)**
Includes limited follow-up care only; does not include future rebasing/relining procedure(s).

D5225   **maxillary partial denture – flexible base (including any clasps, rests and teeth)**

D5226   **mandibular partial denture – flexible base (including any clasps, rests and teeth)**

D5281   **removable unilateral partial denture – one piece cast metal (including clasps and teeth)**

Adjustments to Dentures

D5410   **adjust complete denture – maxillary**

D5411   **adjust complete denture – mandibular**

D5421   **adjust partial denture – maxillary**

D5422   **adjust partial denture – mandibular**

Repairs to Complete Dentures

- **D5511** **repair broken complete denture base, mandibular**

- **D5512** **repair broken complete denture base, maxillary**

  D5520 **replace missing or broken teeth – complete denture (each tooth)**

Repairs to Partial Dentures

- **D5611** **repair resin partial denture base, mandibular**

- **D5612** **repair resin partial denture base, maxillary**

- **D5621** **repair cast partial framework, mandibular**

- **D5622** **repair cast partial framework, maxillary**

  D5630 **repair or replace broken clasp – per tooth**

  D5640 **replace broken teeth – per tooth**

  D5650 **add tooth to existing partial denture**

  D5660 **add clasp to existing partial denture – per tooth**

  D5670 **replace all teeth and acrylic on cast metal framework (maxillary)**

  D5671 **replace all teeth and acrylic on cast metal framework (mandibular)**

Denture Rebase Procedures

Rebase – process of refitting a denture by replacing the base material.

  D5710 **rebase complete maxillary denture**

  D5711 **rebase complete mandibular denture**

  D5720 **rebase maxillary partial denture**

  D5721 **rebase mandibular partial denture**

Denture Reline Procedures

Reline is the process of resurfacing the tissue side of a denture with new base material.

D5730 reline complete maxillary denture (chairside)

D5731 reline complete mandibular denture (chairside)

D5740 reline maxillary partial denture (chairside)

D5741 reline mandibular partial denture (chairside)

D5750 reline complete maxillary denture (laboratory)

D5751 reline complete mandibular denture (laboratory)

D5760 reline maxillary partial denture (laboratory)

D5761 reline mandibular partial denture (laboratory)

Interim Prosthesis

A provisional prosthesis designed for use over a limited period of time, after which it is to be replaced by a more definitive restoration.

D5810 interim complete denture (maxillary)

D5811 interim complete denture (mandibular)

D5820 interim partial denture (maxillary)
Includes any necessary clasps and rests.

D5821 interim partial denture (mandibular)
Includes any necessary clasps and rests.

     ● new procedure code   ▲ revision to a nomenclature or descriptor

Other Removable Prosthetic Services

D5850 tissue conditioning, maxillary
Treatment reline using materials designed to heal unhealthy ridges prior to more definitive final restoration.

D5851 tissue conditioning, mandibular
Treatment reline using materials designed to heal unhealthy ridges prior to more definitive final restoration.

D5862 precision attachment, by report
Each set of male and female components should be reported as one precision attachment. Describe the type of attachment used.

D5863 overdenture – complete maxillary

D5864 overdenture – partial maxillary

D5865 overdenture – complete mandibular

D5866 overdenture – partial mandibular

D5867 replacement of replaceable part of semi-precision or precision attachment (male or female component)

D5875 modification of removable prosthesis following implant surgery
Attachment assemblies are reported using separate codes.

D5899 unspecified removable prosthodontic procedure, by report
Use for a procedure that is not adequately described by a code. Describe procedure.

D5900-D5999 VII. Maxillofacial Prosthetics

D5992 **adjust maxillofacial prosthetic appliance, by report**

D5993 **maintenance and cleaning of a maxillofacial prosthesis (extra- or intra-oral) other than required adjustments, by report**

D5914 **auricular prosthesis**
Synonymous terminology: artificial ear, ear prosthesis.

A removable prosthesis, which artificially restores part or all of the natural ear. Usually, replacement prostheses can be made from the original mold if tissue bed changes have not occurred. Creation of an auricular prosthesis requires fabrication of a mold, from which additional prostheses usually can be made, as needed later (auricular prosthesis, replacement).

D5927 **auricular prosthesis, replacement**
Synonymous terminology: replacement ear.

An artificial ear produced from a previously made mold. A replacement prosthesis does not require fabrication of a new mold. Generally, several prostheses can be made from the same mold assuming no changes occur in the tissue bed due to surgery or age related topographical variations.

D5987 **commissure splint**
Synonymous terminology: lip splint.

A device placed between the lips, which assists in achieving increased opening between the lips. Use of such devices enhances opening where surgical, chemical or electrical alterations of the lips has resulted in severe restriction or contractures.

D5924 **cranial prosthesis**
Synonymous terminology: Skull plate, cranioplasty prosthesis, cranial implant.

A biocompatible, permanently implanted replacement of a portion of the skull bones; an artificial replacement for a portion of the skull bone.

D5925   facial augmentation implant prosthesis
Synonymous terminology: facial implant.

An implantable biocompatible material generally onlayed upon an existing bony area beneath the skin tissue to fill in or collectively raise portions of the overlaying facial skin tissues to create acceptable contours.

Although some forms of pre-made surgical implants are commercially available, the facial augmentation is usually custom made for surgical implantation for each individual patient due to the irregular or extensive nature of the facial deficit.

D5912   facial moulage (complete)
Synonymous terminology: facial impression, face mask impression.

A complete facial moulage impression is a procedure used to record the soft tissue contours of the whole face. The impression is utilized to create a facial moulage and generally is not reusable.

D5911   facial moulage (sectional)
A sectional facial moulage impression is a procedure used to record the soft tissue contours of a portion of the face. Occasionally several separate sectional impressions are made, and then reassembled to provide a full facial contour cast. The impression is utilized to create a partial facial moulage and generally is not reusable.

D5919   facial prosthesis
Synonymous terminology: prosthetic dressing.

A removable prosthesis, which artificially replaces a portion of the face, lost due to surgery, trauma or congenital absence.

Flexion of natural tissues may preclude adaptation and movement of the prosthesis to match the adjacent skin. Salivary leakage, when communicating with the oral cavity, adversely affects retention.

D5929   facial prosthesis, replacement
A replacement facial prosthesis made from the original mold. A replacement prosthesis does not require fabrication of a new mold. Generally, several prostheses can be made from the same mold assuming no changes occur in the tissue bed due to further surgery or age related topographical variations.

● new procedure code   ▲ revision to a nomenclature or descriptor

D5951 **feeding aid**

Synonymous terminology: feeding prosthesis.

A prosthesis, which maintains the right and left maxillary segments of an infant cleft palate patient in their proper orientation until surgery is performed to repair the cleft. It closes the oral-nasal cavity defect, thus enhancing sucking and swallowing.

Used on an interim basis, this prosthesis achieves separation of the oral and nasal cavities in infants born with wide clefts necessitating delayed closure. It is eliminated if surgical closure can be effected or, alternatively, with eruption of the deciduous dentition a pediatric speech aid may be made to facilitate closure of the defect.

D5934 **mandibular resection prosthesis with guide flange**

Synonymous terminology: resection device, resection appliance.

A prosthesis which guides the remaining portion of the mandible, left after a partial resection, into a more normal relationship with the maxilla. This allows for some tooth-to-tooth or an improved tooth contact. It may also artificially replace missing teeth and thereby increase masticatory efficiency.

D5935 **mandibular resection prosthesis without guide flange**

A prosthesis which helps guide the partially resected mandible to a more normal relation with the maxilla allowing for increased tooth contact. It does not have a flange or ramp, however, to assist in directional closure. It may replace missing teeth and thereby increase masticatory efficiency.

Dentists who treat mandibulectomy patients may prefer to replace some, all or none of the teeth in the defect area. Frequently, the defect's margins preclude even partial replacement. Use of a guide (a mandibular resection prosthesis with a guide flange) may not be possible due to anatomical limitations or poor patient tolerance. Ramps, extended occlusal arrangements and irregular occlusal positioning relative to the denture foundation frequently preclude stability of the prostheses, and thus some prostheses are poorly tolerated under such adverse circumstances.

D5913 nasal prosthesis
Synonymous terminology: artificial nose.

A removable prosthesis attached to the skin, which artificially restores part or all of the nose. Fabrication of a nasal prosthesis requires creation of an original mold. Additional prostheses usually can be made from the same mold, and assuming no further tissue changes occur, the same mold can be utilized for extended periods of time.

When a new prosthesis is made from the existing mold, this procedure is termed a nasal prosthesis replacement.

D5926 nasal prosthesis, replacement
Synonymous terminology: replacement nose.

An artificial nose produced from a previously made mold. A replacement prosthesis does not require fabrication of a new mold. Generally, several prostheses can be made from the same mold assuming no changes occur in the tissue bed due to surgery or age related topographical variations.

D5922 nasal septal prosthesis
Synonymous terminology: Septal plug, septal button.

Removable prosthesis to occlude (obturate) a hole within the nasal septal wall. Adverse chemical degradation in this moist environment may require frequent replacement. Silicone prostheses are occasionally subject to fungal invasion.

D5932 obturator prosthesis, definitive
Synonymous terminology: obturator

A prosthesis, which artificially replaces part or all of the maxilla and associated teeth, lost due to surgery, trauma or congenital defects.

A definitive obturator is made when it is deemed that further tissue changes or recurrence of tumor are unlikely and a more permanent prosthetic rehabilitation can be achieved; it is intended for long-term use.

● new procedure code   ▲ revision to a nomenclature or descriptor

D5936   obturator prosthesis, interim

Synonymous terminology: immediate postoperative obturator.

A prosthesis which is made following completion of the initial healing after a surgical resection of a portion or all of one or both the maxillae; frequently many or all teeth in the defect area are replaced by this prosthesis. This prosthesis replaces the surgical obturator, which is usually inserted at, or immediately following the resection.

Generally, an interim obturator is made to facilitate closure of the resultant defect after initial healing has been completed. Unlike the surgical obturator, which usually is made prior to surgery and frequently revised in the operating room during surgery, the interim obturator is made when the defect margins are clearly defined and further surgical revisions are not planned. It is a provisional prosthesis, which may replace some or all lost teeth, and other lost bone and soft tissue structures. Also, it frequently must be revised (termed an obturator prosthesis modification) during subsequent dental procedures (e.g., restorations, gingival surgery) as well as to compensate for further tissue shrinkage before a definitive obturator prosthesis is made.

D5933   obturator prosthesis, modification

Synonymous terminology: adjustment, denture adjustment, temporary or office reline.

Revision or alteration of an existing obturator (surgical, interim, or definitive); possible modifications include relief of the denture base due to tissue compression, augmentation of the seal or peripheral areas to effect adequate sealing or separation between the nasal and oral cavities.

D5931   obturator prosthesis, surgical

Synonymous terminology: Obturator, surgical stayplate, immediate temporary obturator.

A temporary prosthesis inserted during or immediately following surgical or traumatic loss of a portion or all of one or both maxillary bones and contiguous alveolar structures (e.g., gingival tissue, teeth).

Frequent revisions of surgical obturators are necessary during the ensuing healing phase (approximately six months). Some dentists prefer to replace many or all teeth removed by the surgical procedure in the surgical obturator, while others do not replace any teeth. Further surgical revisions may require fabrication of another surgical obturator (e.g., an initially planned small defect may be revised and greatly enlarged after the final pathology report indicates margins are not free of tumor).

D5916 ocular prosthesis
Synonymous terminology: artificial eye, glass eye.

A prosthesis, which artificially replaces an eye missing as a result of trauma, surgery or congenital absence. The prosthesis does not replace missing eyelids or adjacent skin, mucosa or muscle.

Ocular prostheses require semiannual or annual cleaning and polishing. Also, occasional revisions to re-adapt the prosthesis to the tissue bed may be necessary. Glass eyes are rarely made and cannot be re-adapted.

D5923 ocular prosthesis, interim
Synonymous terminology: Eye shell, shell, ocular conformer, conformer.

A temporary replacement generally made of clear acrylic resin for an eye lost due to surgery or trauma. No attempt is made to re-establish esthetics. Fabrication of an interim ocular prosthesis generally implies subsequent fabrication of an aesthetic ocular prosthesis.

D5915 orbital prosthesis
A prosthesis, which artificially restores the eye, eyelids, and adjacent hard and soft tissue, lost as a result of trauma or surgery.

Fabrication of an orbital prosthesis requires creation of an original mold. Additional prostheses usually can be made from the same mold, and assuming no further tissue changes occur, the same mold can be utilized for extended periods of time.

When a new prosthesis is made from the existing mold, this procedure is termed an orbital prosthesis replacement.

D5928 orbital prosthesis, replacement
A replacement for a previously made orbital prosthesis. A replacement prosthesis does not require fabrication of a new mold. Generally, several prostheses can be made from the same mold assuming no changes occur in the tissue bed due to surgery or age related topographical variations.

D5954 palatal augmentation prosthesis
Synonymous terminology: superimposed prosthesis, maxillary glossectomy prosthesis, maxillary speech prosthesis, palatal drop prosthesis.

A removable prosthesis which alters the hard and/or soft palate's topographical form adjacent to the tongue.

D5955 palatal lift prosthesis, definitive
A prosthesis which elevates the soft palate superiorly and aids in restoration of soft palate functions which may be lost due to an acquired, congenital or developmental defect.

A definitive palatal lift is usually made for patients whose experience with an interim palatal lift has been successful, especially if surgical alterations are deemed unwarranted.

D5958 palatal lift prosthesis, interim
Synonymous terminology: diagnostic palatal lift.

A prosthesis which elevates and assists in restoring soft palate function which may be lost due to clefting, surgery, trauma or unknown paralysis. It is intended for interim use to determine its usefulness in achieving palatalpharyngeal competency or enhance swallowing reflexes.

This prosthesis is intended for interim use as a diagnostic aid to assess the level of possible improvement in speech intelligibility. Some clinicians believe use of a palatal lift on an interim basis may stimulate an otherwise flaccid soft palate to increase functional activity, subsequently lessening its need.

D5959 palatal lift prosthesis, modification
Synonymous terminology: revision of lift, adjustment.

Alterations in the adaptation, contour, form or function of an existing palatal lift necessitated due to tissue impingement, lack of function, poor clasp adaptation or the like.

D5985 radiation cone locator
Synonymous terminology: docking device, cone locator.

A prosthesis utilized to direct and reduplicate the path of radiation to an oral tumor during a split course of irradiation.

D5984 radiation shield
Synonymous terminology: radiation stent, tongue protector, lead shield.

An intraoral prosthesis designed to shield adjacent tissues from radiation during orthovoltage treatment of malignant lesions of the head and neck region.

D5953 speech aid prosthesis, adult
Synonymous terminology: prosthetic speech appliance, speech aid, speech bulb.

A definitive prosthesis, which can improve speech in adult cleft palate patients either by obturating (sealing off) a palatal cleft or fistula, or occasionally by assisting an incompetent soft palate. Both mechanisms are necessary to achieve velopharyngeal competency.

Generally, this prosthesis is fabricated when no further growth is anticipated and the objective is to achieve long-term use. Hence, more precise materials and techniques are utilized. Occasionally such procedures are accomplished in conjunction with precision attachments in crown work undertaken on some or all maxillary teeth to achieve improved aesthetics.

D5960 speech aid prosthesis, modification
Synonymous terminology: adjustment, repair, revision.

Any revision of a pediatric or adult speech aid not necessitating its replacement.

Frequently, revisions of the obturating section of any speech aid are required to facilitate enhanced speech intelligibility. Such revisions or repairs do not require complete remaking of the prosthesis, thus extending its longevity.

D5952 speech aid prosthesis, pediatric
Synonymous terminology: nasopharyngeal obturator, speech appliance, obturator, cleft palate appliance, prosthetic speech aid, speech bulb.

A temporary or interim prosthesis used to close a defect in the hard and/or soft palate. It may replace tissue lost due to developmental or surgical alterations. It is necessary for the production of intelligible speech.

Normal lateral growth of the palatal bones necessitates occasional replacement of this prosthesis. Intermittent revisions of the obturator section can assist in maintenance of palatalpharyngeal closure (termed a speech aid prosthesis modification). Frequently, such prostheses are not fabricated before the deciduous dentition is fully erupted since clasp retention is often essential.

D5988 surgical splint

Synonymous terminology: Gunning splint, modified Gunning splint, labiolingual splint, fenestrated splint, Kingsley splint, cast metal splint.

Splints are designed to utilize existing teeth and/or alveolar processes as points of anchorage to assist in stabilization and immobilization of broken bones during healing. They are used to re-establish, as much as possible, normal occlusal relationships during the process of immobilization. Frequently, existing prostheses (e.g., a patient's complete dentures) can be modified to serve as surgical splints. Frequently, surgical splints have arch bars added to facilitate intermaxillary fixation. Rubber elastics may be used to assist in this process. Circummandibular eyelet hooks can be utilized for enhanced stabilization with wiring to adjacent bone.

D5982 surgical stent

Synonymous terminology: periodontal stent, skin graft stent, columellar stent.

Stents are utilized to apply pressure to soft tissues to facilitate healing and prevent cicatrization or collapse.

A surgical stent may be required in surgical and post-surgical revisions to achieve close approximation of tissues. Usually such materials as temporary or interim soft denture liners, gutta percha, or dental modeling impression compound may be used.

D5937 trismus appliance (not for TMD treatment)

Synonymous terminology: occlusal device for mandibular trismus, dynamic bite opener.

A prosthesis, which assists the patient in increasing their oral aperture width in order to eat as well as maintain oral hygiene.

Several versions and designs are possible, all intending to ease the severe lack of oral opening experienced by many patients immediately following extensive intraoral surgical procedures.

Carriers

D5986 fluoride gel carrier

Synonymous terminology: fluoride applicator.

A prosthesis, which covers the teeth in either dental arch and is used to apply topical fluoride in close proximity to tooth enamel and dentin for several minutes daily.

D5994 periodontal medicament carrier with peripheral seal – laboratory processed

A custom fabricated, laboratory processed carrier that covers the teeth and alveolar mucosa. Used as a vehicle to deliver prescribed medicaments for sustained contact with the gingiva, alveolar mucosa, and into the periodontal sulcus or pocket.

D5983 radiation carrier

Synonymous terminology: radiotherapy prosthesis, carrier prosthesis, radiation applicator, radium carrier, intracavity carrier, intracavity applicator.

A device used to administer radiation to confined areas by means of capsules, beads or needles of radiation emitting materials such as radium or cesium. Its function is to hold the radiation source securely in the same location during the entire period of treatment.

Radiation oncologists occasionally request these devices to achieve close approximation and controlled application of radiation to a tumor deemed amiable to eradication.

D5991 vesiculobullous disease medicament carrier

A custom fabricated carrier that covers the teeth and alveolar mucosa, or alveolar mucosa alone, and is used to deliver prescription medicaments for treatment of immunologically mediated vesiculobullous diseases.

D5999 unspecified maxillofacial prosthesis, by report

Used for procedure that is not adequately described by a code. Describe procedure.

D6000-D6199 VIII. Implant Services

Local anesthesia is usually considered to be part of Implant Services procedures.

Pre-Surgical Services

D6190 radiographic/surgical implant index, by report
An appliance, designed to relate osteotomy or fixture position to existing anatomic structures, to be utilized during radiographic exposure for treatment planning and/or during osteotomy creation for fixture installation.

Surgical Services

Report surgical implant procedure using codes in this section.

D6010 surgical placement of implant body: endosteal implant

D6011 second stage implant surgery
Surgical access to an implant body for placement of a healing cap or to enable placement of an abutment.

D6012 surgical placement of interim implant body for transitional prosthesis: endosteal implant
Includes removal during later therapy to accommodate the definitive restoration, which may include placement of other implants.

D6013 surgical placement of mini implant

D6040 surgical placement: eposteal implant
An eposteal (subperiosteal) framework of a biocompatible material designed and fabricated to fit on the surface of the bone of the mandible or maxilla with permucosal extensions which provide support and attachment of a prosthesis. This may be a complete arch or unilateral appliance. Eposteal implants rest upon the bone and under the periosteum.

D6050 **surgical placement: transosteal implant**
A transosteal (transosseous) biocompatible device with threaded posts penetrating both the superior and inferior cortical bone plates of the mandibular symphysis and exiting through the permucosa providing support and attachment for a dental prosthesis. Transosteal implants are placed completely through the bone and into the oral cavity from extraoral or intraoral.

D6100 **implant removal, by report**
This procedure involves the surgical removal of an implant. Describe procedure.

D6101 **debridement of a peri-implant defect or defects surrounding a single implant, and surface cleaning of the exposed implant surfaces, including flap entry and closure**

D6102 **debridement and osseous contouring of a peri-implant defect or defects surrounding a single implant and includes surface cleaning of the exposed implant surfaces, including flap entry and closure**

D6103 **bone graft for repair of peri-implant defect – does not include flap entry and closure**
Placement of a barrier membrane or biologic materials to aid in osseous regeneration, are reported separately.

D6104 **bone graft at time of implant placement**
Placement of a barrier membrane, or biologic materials to aid in osseous regeneration are reported separately.

Implant Supported Prosthetics

Supporting Structures

D6055 connecting bar – implant supported or abutment supported
Utilized to stabilize and anchor a prosthesis.

D6056 prefabricated abutment – includes modification and placement
Modification of a prefabricated abutment may be necessary.

D6057 custom fabricated abutment – includes placement
Created by a laboratory process, specific for an individual application.

D6051 interim abutment
Includes placement and removal. A healing cap is not an interim abutment.

D6052 semi-precision attachment abutment
Includes placement of keeper assembly.

Implant/Abutment Supported Removable Dentures

D6110 implant /abutment supported removable denture for edentulous arch – maxillary

D6111 implant /abutment supported removable denture for edentulous arch – mandibular

D6112 implant /abutment supported removable denture for partially edentulous arch – maxillary

D6113 implant /abutment supported removable denture for partially edentulous arch – mandibular

Implant/Abutment Supported Fixed Dentures (Hybrid Prosthesis)

D6114 implant /abutment supported fixed denture for edentulous arch – maxillary

D6115 implant /abutment supported fixed denture for edentulous arch – mandibular

D6116 implant /abutment supported fixed denture for partially edentulous arch – maxillary

D6117 **implant /abutment supported fixed denture for partially edentulous arch – mandibular**

• **D6118** **implant/abutment supported interim fixed denture for edentulous arch – mandibular**
Used when a period of healing is necessary prior to fabrication and placement of a permanent prosthetic.

• **D6119** **implant/abutment supported interim fixed denture for edentulous arch – maxillary**
Used when a period of healing is necessary prior to fabrication and placement of a permanent prosthetic.

Single Crowns, Abutment Supported

D6058 **abutment supported porcelain/ceramic crown**
A single crown restoration that is retained, supported and stabilized by an abutment on an implant.

D6059 **abutment supported porcelain fused to metal crown (high noble metal)**
A single metal-ceramic crown restoration that is retained, supported and stabilized by an abutment on an implant.

D6060 **abutment supported porcelain fused to metal crown (predominantly base metal)**
A single metal-ceramic crown restoration that is retained, supported and stabilized by an abutment on an implant.

D6061 **abutment supported porcelain fused to metal crown (noble metal)**
A single metal-ceramic crown restoration that is retained, supported and stabilized by an abutment on an implant.

D6062 **abutment supported cast metal crown (high noble metal)**
A single cast metal crown restoration that is retained, supported and stabilized by an abutment on an implant.

D6063 **abutment supported cast metal crown (predominantly base metal)**
A single cast metal crown restoration that is retained, supported and stabilized by an abutment on an implant.

D6064 abutment supported cast metal crown (noble metal)
A single cast metal crown restoration that is retained, supported and stabilized by an abutment on an implant.

D6094 abutment supported crown (titanium)
A single crown restoration that is retained, supported and stabilized by an abutment on an implant. May be cast or milled.

Single Crowns, Implant Supported

D6065 implant supported porcelain/ceramic crown
A single crown restoration that is retained, supported and stabilized by an implant.

D6066 implant supported porcelain fused to metal crown (titanium, titanium alloy, high noble metal)
A single metal-ceramic crown restoration that is retained, supported and stabilized by an implant.

D6067 implant supported metal crown (titanium, titanium alloy, high noble metal)
A single cast metal or milled crown restoration that is retained, supported and stabilized by an implant.

Fixed Partial Denture Retainer, Abutment Supported

D6068 abutment supported retainer for porcelain/ceramic FPD
A ceramic retainer for a fixed partial denture that gains retention, support and stability from an abutment on an implant.

D6069 abutment supported retainer for porcelain fused to metal FPD (high noble metal)
A metal-ceramic retainer for a fixed partial denture that gains retention, support and stability from an abutment on an implant.

D6070 abutment supported retainer for porcelain fused to metal FPD (predominantly base metal)
A metal-ceramic retainer for a fixed partial denture that gains retention, support and stability from an abutment on an implant.

D6071 abutment supported retainer for porcelain fused to metal FPD (noble metal)
A metal-ceramic retainer for a fixed partial denture that gains retention, support and stability from an abutment on an implant.

D6072 abutment supported retainer for cast metal FPD (high noble metal)
A cast metal retainer for a fixed partial denture that gains retention, support and stability from an abutment on an implant.

D6073 abutment supported retainer for cast metal FPD (predominantly base metal)
A cast metal retainer for a fixed partial denture that gains retention, support and stability from an abutment on an implant.

D6074 abutment supported retainer for cast metal FPD (noble metal)
A cast metal retainer for a fixed partial denture that gains retention, support and stability from an abutment on an implant.

D6194 abutment supported retainer crown for FPD (titanium)
A retainer for a fixed partial denture that gains retention, support and stability from an abutment on an implant. May be cast or milled.

Fixed Partial Denture Retainer, Implant Supported

D6075 implant supported retainer for ceramic FPD
A ceramic retainer for a fixed partial denture that gains retention, support and stability from an implant.

D6076 implant supported retainer for porcelain fused to metal FPD (titanium, titanium alloy, or high noble metal)
A metal-ceramic retainer for a fixed partial denture that gains retention, support and stability from an implant.

D6077 implant supported retainer for cast metal FPD (titanium, titanium alloy, or high noble metal)
A cast metal retainer for a fixed partial denture that gains retention, support and stability from an implant.

Other Implant Services

D6080 **implant maintenance procedures when prostheses are removed and reinserted, including cleansing of prostheses and abutments**
This procedure includes active debriding of the implant(s) and examination of all aspects of the implant system(s), including the occlusion and stability of the superstructure. The patient is also instructed in thorough daily cleansing of the implant(s). This is not a per implant code, and is indicated for implant supported fixed prostheses.

▲ **D6081** **scaling and debridement in the presence of inflammation or mucositis of a single implant, including cleaning of the implant surfaces, without flap entry and closure**
This procedure is not performed in conjunction with D1110, D4910, or D4346.

D6085 **provisional implant crown**
Used when a period of healing is necessary prior to fabrication and placement of permanent prosthetic.

D6090 **repair implant supported prosthesis, by report**
This procedure involves the repair or replacement of any part of the implant supported prosthesis.

D6091 **replacement of semi-precision or precision attachment (male or female component) of implant/abutment supported prosthesis, per attachment**
This procedure applies to the replaceable male or female component of the attachment.

D6092 **re-cement or re-bond implant/abutment supported crown**

D6093 **re-cement or re-bond implant/abutment supported fixed partial denture**

D6095 **repair implant abutment, by report**
This procedure involves the repair or replacement of any part of the implant abutment.

• **D6096** **remove broken implant retaining screw**

D6199   **unspecified implant procedure, by report**
Use for procedure that is not adequately described by a code.
Describe procedure.

● new procedure code   ▲ revision to a nomenclature or descriptor

D6200–D6999   IX. Prosthodontics, fixed

Each retainer and each pontic constitutes a unit in a fixed partial denture.

Local anesthesia is usually considered to be part of Fixed Prosthodontic procedures.

The term "fixed partial denture" or FPD is synonymous with fixed bridge or bridgework.

Fixed partial denture prosthetic procedures include routine temporary prosthetics. When indicated, interim or provisional codes should be reported separately.

Fixed Partial Denture Pontics

D6205   pontic – indirect resin based composite
Not to be used as a temporary or provisional prosthesis.

D6210   pontic – cast high noble metal

D6211   pontic – cast predominantly base metal

D6212   pontic – cast noble metal

D6214   pontic – titanium

D6240   pontic – porcelain fused to high noble metal

D6241   pontic – porcelain fused to predominantly base metal

D6242   pontic – porcelain fused to noble metal

D6245   pontic – porcelain/ceramic

D6250   pontic – resin with high noble metal

D6251   pontic – resin with predominantly base metal

D6252   pontic – resin with noble metal

D6253   provisional pontic– further treatment or completion of diagnosis necessary prior to final impression
Not to be used as a temporary pontic for routine prosthetic fixed partial dentures.

Fixed Partial Denture Retainers – Inlays/Onlays

D6545 retainer – cast metal for resin bonded fixed prosthesis

D6548 retainer – porcelain/ceramic for resin bonded fixed prosthesis

D6549 resin retainer – for resin bonded fixed prosthesis

D6600 retainer inlay – porcelain/ceramic, two surfaces

D6601 retainer inlay – porcelain/ceramic, three or more surfaces

D6602 retainer inlay – cast high noble metal, two surfaces

D6603 retainer inlay – cast high noble metal, three or more surfaces

D6604 retainer inlay – cast predominantly base metal, two surfaces

D6605 retainer inlay – cast predominantly base metal, three or more surfaces

D6606 retainer inlay – cast noble metal, two surfaces

D6607 retainer inlay – cast noble metal, three or more surfaces

D6624 retainer inlay – titanium

D6608 retainer onlay – porcelain/ceramic, two surfaces

D6609 retainer onlay – porcelain/ceramic, three or more surfaces

D6610 retainer onlay – cast high noble metal, two surfaces

D6611 retainer onlay – cast high noble metal, three or more surfaces

D6612 retainer onlay – cast predominantly base metal, two surfaces

D6613 retainer onlay – cast predominantly base metal, three or more surfaces

D6614 retainer onlay – cast noble metal, two surfaces

D6615 retainer onlay – cast noble metal, three or more surfaces

D6634 retainer onlay – titanium

Fixed Partial Denture Retainers – Crowns

D6710 retainer crown – indirect resin based composite
Not to be used as a temporary or provisional prosthesis.

D6720 retainer crown – resin with high noble metal

D6721 retainer crown – resin with predominantly base metal

D6722 retainer crown – resin with noble metal

D6740 retainer crown – porcelain/ceramic

D6750 retainer crown – porcelain fused to high noble metal

D6751 retainer crown – porcelain fused to predominantly base metal

D6752 retainer crown – porcelain fused to noble metal

D6780 retainer crown – ¾ cast high noble metal

D6781 retainer crown – ¾ cast predominantly base metal

D6782 retainer crown – ¾ cast noble metal

D6783 retainer crown – ¾ porcelain/ceramic

D6790 retainer crown – full cast high noble metal

D6791 retainer crown – full cast predominantly base metal

D6792 retainer crown – full cast noble metal

D6794 retainer crown – titanium

D6793 provisional retainer crown– further treatment or completion of diagnosis necessary prior to final impression
Not to be used as a temporary retainer crown for routine prosthetic fixed partial dentures.

Other Fixed Partial Denture Services

D6920 connector bar
A device attached to fixed partial denture retainer or coping which serves to stabilize and anchor a removable overdenture prosthesis.

D6930 re-cement or re-bond fixed partial denture

D6940 stress breaker
A non-rigid connector.

D6950 precision attachment
A male and female pair constitutes one precision attachment, and is separate from the prosthesis.

D6980 fixed partial denture repair necessitated by restorative material failure

D6985 pediatric partial denture, fixed
This prosthesis is used primarily for aesthetic purposes.

D6999 unspecified fixed prosthodontic procedure, by report
Used for procedure that is not adequately described by a code. Describe procedure.

D7000-D7999 X. Oral and Maxillofacial Surgery

Local anesthesia is usually considered to be part of Oral and Maxillofacial Surgical procedures.

For dental benefit reporting purposes a quadrant is defined as four or more contiguous teeth and/or teeth spaces distal to the midline.

Extractions (Includes Local Anesthesia, Suturing If Needed, and Routine Postoperative Care)

▲ **D7111** **extraction, coronal remnants – primary tooth**
Removal of soft tissue-retained coronal remnants.

D7140 **extraction, erupted tooth or exposed root (elevation and/or forceps removal)**
Includes removal of tooth structure, minor smoothing of socket bone, and closure, as necessary.

D7210 **extraction, erupted tooth requiring removal of bone and/ or sectioning of tooth, and including elevation of mucoperiosteal flap if indicated**
Includes related cutting of gingiva and bone, removal of tooth structure, minor smoothing of socket bone and closure.

D7220 **removal of impacted tooth – soft tissue**
Occlusal surface of tooth covered by soft tissue; requires mucoperiosteal flap elevation.

D7230 **removal of impacted tooth – partially bony**
Part of crown covered by bone; requires mucoperiosteal flap elevation and bone removal.

D7240 **removal of impacted tooth – completely bony**
Most or all of crown covered by bone; requires mucoperiosteal flap elevation and bone removal.

D7241 **removal of impacted tooth – completely bony, with unusual surgical complications**
Most or all of crown covered by bone; unusually difficult or complicated due to factors such as nerve dissection required, separate closure of maxillary sinus required or aberrant tooth position.

D7250 **removal of residual tooth roots (cutting procedure)**
Includes cutting of soft tissue and bone, removal of tooth structure, and closure.

D7251 **coronectomy – intentional partial tooth removal**
Intentional partial tooth removal is performed when a neurovascular complication is likely if the entire impacted tooth is removed.

Other Surgical Procedures

D7260 **oroantral fistula closure**
Excision of fistulous tract between maxillary sinus and oral cavity and closure by advancement flap.

D7261 **primary closure of a sinus perforation**
Subsequent to surgical removal of tooth, exposure of sinus requiring repair, or immediate closure of oroantral or oralnasal communication in absence of fistulous tract.

D7270 **tooth re-implantation and/or stabilization of accidentally evulsed or displaced tooth**
Includes splinting and/or stabilization.

D7272 **tooth transplantation (includes re-implantation from one site to another and splinting and/or stabilization)**

D7280 **exposure of an unerupted tooth**
An incision is made and the tissue is reflected and bone removed as necessary to expose the crown of an impacted tooth not intended to be extracted.

D7282 **mobilization of erupted or malpositioned tooth to aid eruption**
To move/luxate teeth to eliminate ankylosis; not in conjunction with an extraction.

D7283 **placement of device to facilitate eruption of impacted tooth**
Placement of an orthodontic bracket, band or other device on an unerupted tooth, after its exposure, to aid in its eruption. Report the surgical exposure separately using D7280.

● new procedure code   ▲ revision to a nomenclature or descriptor

D7285 incisional biopsy of oral tissue – hard (bone, tooth)
For partial removal of specimen only. This procedure involves biopsy of osseous lesions and is not used for apicoectomy/periradicular surgery. This procedure does not entail an excision.

D7286 incisional biopsy of oral tissue – soft
For partial removal of an architecturally intact specimen only. This procedure is not used at the same time as codes for apicoectomy/periradicular curettage. This procedure does not entail an excision.

D7287 exfoliative cytological sample collection
For collection of non-transepithelial cytology sample via mild scraping of the oral mucosa.

D7288 brush biopsy – transepithelial sample collection
For collection of oral disaggregated transepithelial cells via rotational brushing of the oral mucosa.

D7290 surgical repositioning of teeth
Grafting procedure(s) is/are additional.

D7291 transseptal fiberotomy/supra crestal fiberotomy, by report
The supraosseous connective tissue attachment is surgically severed around the involved teeth. Where there are adjacent teeth, the transseptal fiberotomy of a single tooth will involve a minimum of three teeth. Since the incisions are within the gingival sulcus and tissue and the root surface is not instrumented, this procedure heals by the reunion of connective tissue with the root surface on which viable periodontal tissue is present (reattachment).

D7292 placement of temporary anchorage device [screw retained plate] requiring flap; includes device removal

D7293 placement of temporary anchorage device requiring flap; includes device removal

D7294 placement of temporary anchorage device without flap; includes device removal

D7295 harvest of bone for use in autogenous grafting procedure
Reported in addition to those autogenous graft placement procedures that do not include harvesting of bone.

- **D7296 corticotomy – one to three teeth or tooth spaces, per quadrant**
  This procedure involves creating multiple cuts, perforations, or removal of cortical, alveolar or basal bone of the jaw for the purpose of facilitating orthodontic repositioning of the dentition. This procedure includes flap entry and closure. Graft material and membrane, if used, should be reported separately.

- **D7297 corticotomy – four or more teeth or tooth spaces, per quadrant**
  This procedure involves creating multiple cuts, perforations, or removal of cortical, alveolar or basal bone of the jaw for the purpose of facilitating orthodontic repositioning of the dentition. This procedure includes flap entry and closure. Graft material and membrane, if used, should be reported separately.

Alveoloplasty – Preparation of Ridge

D7310 alveoloplasty in conjunction with extractions – four or more teeth or tooth spaces, per quadrant
The alveoloplasty is distinct (separate procedure) from extractions. Usually in preparation for a prosthesis or other treatments such as radiation therapy and transplant surgery.

D7311 alveoloplasty in conjunction with extractions – one to three teeth or tooth spaces, per quadrant
The alveoloplasty is distinct (separate procedure) from extractions. Usually in preparation for a prosthesis or other treatments such as radiation therapy and transplant surgery.

D7320 alveoloplasty not in conjunction with extractions – four or more teeth or tooth spaces, per quadrant
No extractions performed in an edentulous area. See D7310 if teeth are being extracted concurrently with the alveoloplasty. Usually in preparation for a prosthesis or other treatments such as radiation therapy and transplant surgery.

D7321 alveoloplasty not in conjunction with extractions – one to three teeth or tooth spaces, per quadrant
No extractions performed in an edentulous area. See D7311 if teeth are being extracted concurrently with the alveoloplasty. Usually in preparation for a prosthesis or other treatments such as radiation therapy and transplant surgery.

    ● new procedure code   ▲ revision to a nomenclature or descriptor

Vestibuloplasty

Any of a series of surgical procedures designed to increase relative alveolar ridge height.

D7340 **vestibuloplasty – ridge extension (secondary epithelialization)**

D7350 **vestibuloplasty – ridge extension (including soft tissue grafts, muscle reattachment, revision of soft tissue attachment and management of hypertrophied and hyperplastic tissue)**

Excision of Soft Tissue Lesions

Includes non-odontogenic cysts.

D7410 **excision of benign lesion up to 1.25 cm**

D7411 **excision of benign lesion greater than 1.25 cm**

D7412 **excision of benign lesion, complicated**
Requires extensive undermining with advancement or rotational flap closure.

D7413 **excision of malignant lesion up to 1.25 cm**

D7414 **excision of malignant lesion greater than 1.25 cm**

D7415 **excision of malignant lesion, complicated**
Requires extensive undermining with advancement or rotational flap closure.

D7465 **destruction of lesion(s) by physical or chemical method, by report**
Examples include using cryo, laser or electro surgery.

Excision of Intra-Osseous Lesions

D7440 **excision of malignant tumor – lesion diameter up to 1.25 cm**

D7441 **excision of malignant tumor – lesion diameter greater than 1.25 cm**

D7450 **removal of benign odontogenic cyst or tumor – lesion diameter up to 1.25 cm**

D7451 removal of benign odontogenic cyst or tumor – lesion diameter greater than 1.25 cm

D7460 removal of benign nonodontogenic cyst or tumor – lesion diameter up to 1.25 cm

D7461 removal of benign nonodontogenic cyst or tumor – lesion diameter greater than 1.25 cm

Excision of Bone Tissue

D7471 removal of lateral exostosis (maxilla or mandible)

D7472 removal of torus palatinus

D7473 removal of torus mandibularis

D7485 reduction of osseous tuberosity

D7490 radical resection of maxilla or mandible
Partial resection of maxilla or mandible; removal of lesion and defect with margin of normal appearing bone. Reconstruction and bone grafts should be reported separately.

Surgical Incision

D7510 incision and drainage of abscess – intraoral soft tissue
Involves incision through mucosa, including periodontal origins.

D7511 incision and drainage of abscess – intraoral soft tissue – complicated (includes drainage of multiple fascial spaces)
Incision is made intraorally and dissection is extended into adjacent fascial space(s) to provide adequate drainage of abscess/cellulitis.

D7520 incision and drainage of abscess – extraoral soft tissue
Involves incision through skin.

D7521 incision and drainage of abscess – extraoral soft tissue – complicated (includes drainage of multiple fascial spaces)
Incision is made extraorally and dissection is extended into adjacent fascial space(s) to provide adequate drainage of abscess/cellulitis.

D7530 **removal of foreign body from mucosa, skin, or subcutaneous alveolar tissue**

D7540 **removal of reaction producing foreign bodies, musculoskeletal system**
May include, but is not limited to, removal of splinters, pieces of wire, etc., from muscle and/or bone.

D7550 **partial ostectomy/sequestrectomy for removal of non-vital bone**
Removal of loose or sloughed-off dead bone caused by infection or reduced blood supply.

D7560 **maxillary sinusotomy for removal of tooth fragment or foreign body**

Treatment of Closed Fractures

D7610 **maxilla – open reduction (teeth immobilized, if present)**
Teeth may be wired, banded or splinted together to prevent movement. Incision required for interosseous fixation.

D7620 **maxilla – closed reduction (teeth immobilized, if present)**
No incision required to reduce fracture. See D7610 if interosseous fixation is applied.

D7630 **mandible – open reduction (teeth immobilized, if present)**
Teeth may be wired, banded or splinted together to prevent movement. Incision required to reduce fracture.

D7640 **mandible – closed reduction (teeth immobilized, if present)**
No incision required to reduce fracture. See D7630 if interosseous fixation is applied.

D7650 **malar and/or zygomatic arch – open reduction**

D7660 **malar and/or zygomatic arch – closed reduction**

D7670 **alveolus – closed reduction, may include stabilization of teeth**
Teeth may be wired, banded or splinted together to prevent movement.

D7671 **alveolus – open reduction, may include stabilization of teeth**
Teeth may be wired, banded or splinted together to prevent movement.

D7680 **facial bones – complicated reduction with fixation and multiple surgical approaches**
Facial bones include upper and lower jaw, cheek, and bones around eyes, nose, and ears.

Treatment of Open Fractures

D7710 **maxilla – open reduction**
Incision required to reduce fracture.

D7720 **maxilla – closed reduction**

D7730 **mandible – open reduction**
Incision required to reduce fracture.

D7740 **mandible – closed reduction**

D7750 **malar and/or zygomatic arch – open reduction**
Incision required to reduce fracture.

D7760 **malar and/or zygomatic arch – closed reduction**

D7770 **alveolus – open reduction stabilization of teeth**
Fractured bone(s) are exposed to mouth or outside the face. Incision required to reduce fracture.

D7771 **alveolus, closed reduction stabilization of teeth**
Fractured bone(s) are exposed to mouth or outside the face.

D7780 **facial bones – complicated reduction with fixation and multiple approaches**
Incision required to reduce fracture. Facial bones include upper and lower jaw, cheek, and bones around eyes, nose, and ears.

Reduction of Dislocation and Management of Other Temporomandibular Joint Dysfunctions

Procedures that are an integral part of a primary procedure should not be reported separately.

D7810 **open reduction of dislocation**
Access to TMJ via surgical opening.

D7820 **closed reduction of dislocation**
Joint manipulated into place; no surgical exposure.

D7830 **manipulation under anesthesia**
Usually done under general anesthesia or intravenous sedation.

D7840 **condylectomy**
Removal of all or portion of the mandibular condyle (separate procedure).

D7850 **surgical discectomy, with/without implant**
Excision of the intra-articular disc of a joint.

D7852 **disc repair**
Repositioning and/or sculpting of disc; repair of perforated posterior attachment.

D7854 **synovectomy**
Excision of a portion or all of the synovial membrane of a joint.

D7856 **myotomy**
Cutting of muscle for therapeutic purposes (separate procedure).

D7858 **joint reconstruction**
Reconstruction of osseous components including or excluding soft tissues of the joint with autogenous, homologous, or alloplastic materials.

D7860 **arthrotomy**
Cutting into joint (separate procedure).

D7865 **arthroplasty**
Reduction of osseous components of the joint to create a pseudoarthrosis or eliminate an irregular remodeling pattern (osteophytes).

D7870 arthrocentesis
Withdrawal of fluid from a joint space by aspiration.

D7871 non-arthroscopic lysis and lavage
Inflow and outflow catheters are placed into the joint space. The joint is lavaged and manipulated as indicated in an effort to release minor adhesions and synovial vacuum phenomenon as well as to remove inflammation products from the joint space.

D7872 arthroscopy – diagnosis, with or without biopsy

D7873 arthroscopy: lavage and lysis of adhesions
Removal of adhesions using the arthroscope and lavage of the joint cavities.

D7874 arthroscopy: disc repositioning and stabilization
Repositioning and stabilization of disc using arthroscopic techniques.

D7875 arthroscopy: synovectomy
Removal of inflamed and hyperplastic synovium (partial/complete) via an arthroscopic technique.

D7876 arthroscopy: discectomy
Removal of disc and remodeled posterior attachment via the arthroscope.

D7877 arthroscopy: debridement
Removal of pathologic hard and/or soft tissue using the arthroscope.

D7880 occlusal orthotic device, by report
Presently includes splints provided for treatment of temporomandibular joint dysfunction.

D7881 occlusal orthotic device adjustment

D7899 unspecified TMD therapy, by report
Used for procedure that is not adequately described by a code. Describe procedure.

● new procedure code ▲ revision to a nomenclature or descriptor

Repair of Traumatic Wounds

Excludes closure of surgical incisions.

D7910 suture of recent small wounds up to 5 cm

Complicated Suturing (Reconstruction Requiring Delicate Handling of Tissues and Wide Undermining for Meticulous Closure)

Excludes closure of surgical incisions.

D7911 complicated suture – up to 5 cm

D7912 complicated suture – greater than 5 cm

Other Repair Procedures

D7920 skin graft (identify defect covered, location and type of graft)

D7921 collection and application of autologous blood concentrate product

D7940 osteoplasty – for orthognathic deformities
Reconstruction of jaws for correction of congenital, developmental or acquired traumatic or surgical deformity.

D7941 osteotomy – mandibular rami

D7943 osteotomy – mandibular rami with bone graft; includes obtaining the graft

D7944 osteotomy – segmented or subapical
Report by range of tooth numbers within segment.

D7945 osteotomy – body of mandible
Sectioning of lower jaw. This includes the exposure, bone cut, fixation, routine wound closure and normal post-operative follow-up care.

D7946 LeFort I (maxilla – total)
Sectioning of the upper jaw. This includes exposure, bone cuts, downfracture, repositioning, fixation, routine wound closure and normal post-operative follow-up care.

D7947 LeFort I (maxilla – segmented)
When reporting a surgically assisted palatal expansion without downfracture, this code would entail a reduced service and should be "by report."

D7948 LeFort II or LeFort III (osteoplasty of facial bones for midface hypoplasia or retrusion) – without bone graft
Sectioning of upper jaw. This includes exposure, bone cuts, downfracture, segmentation of maxilla, repositioning, fixation, routine wound closure and normal post-operative follow-up care.

D7949 LeFort II or LeFort III – with bone graft
Includes obtaining autografts.

D7950 osseous, osteoperiosteal, or cartilage graft of the mandible or maxilla – autogenous or nonautogenous, by report
This procedure is for ridge augmentation or reconstruction to increase height, width and/or volume of residual alveolar ridge. It includes obtaining graft material. Placement of a barrier membrane, if used, should be reported separately.

D7951 sinus augmentation with bone or bone substitutes via a lateral open approach
The augmentation of the sinus cavity to increase alveolar height for reconstruction of edentulous portions of the maxilla. This procedure is performed via a lateral open approach. This includes obtaining the bone or bone substitutes. Placement of a barrier membrane if used should be reported separately.

D7952 sinus augmentation via a vertical approach
The augmentation of the sinus to increase alveolar height by vertical access through the ridge crest by raising the floor of the sinus and grafting as necessary. This includes obtaining the bone or bone substitutes.

D7953 bone replacement graft for ridge preservation – per site
Graft is placed in an extraction or implant removal site at the time of

the extraction or removal to preserve ridge integrity (e.g., clinically indicated in preparation for implant reconstruction or where alveolar contour is critical to planned prosthetic reconstruction). Does not include obtaining graft material. Membrane, if used should be reported separately.

D7955 **repair of maxillofacial soft and/or hard tissue defect**
Reconstruction of surgical, traumatic, or congenital defects of the facial bones, including the mandible, may utilize graft materials in conjunction with soft tissue procedures to repair and restore the facial bones to form and function. This does not include obtaining the graft and these procedures may require multiple surgical approaches. This procedure does not include edentulous maxilla and mandibular reconstruction for prosthetic considerations.

D7960 **frenulectomy – also known as frenectomy or frenotomy – separate procedure not incidental to another procedure**
Removal or release of mucosal and muscle elements of a buccal, labial or lingual frenum that is associated with a pathological condition, or interferes with proper oral development or treatment.

D7963 **frenuloplasty**
Excision of frenum with accompanying excision or repositioning of aberrant muscle and z-plasty or other local flap closure.

D7970 **excision of hyperplastic tissue – per arch**

D7971 **excision of pericoronal gingiva**
Removal of inflammatory or hypertrophied tissues surrounding partially erupted/impacted teeth.

D7972 **surgical reduction of fibrous tuberosity**

● **D7979** **non – surgical sialolithotomy**
A sialolith is removed from the gland or ductal portion of the gland without surgical incision into the gland or the duct of the gland; for example via manual manipulation, ductal dilation, or any other non-surgical method.

▲ **D7980** **surgical sialolithotomy**
Procedure by which a stone within a salivary gland or its duct is removed, either intraorally or extraorally.

D7981 excision of salivary gland, by report

D7982 sialodochoplasty
Procedure for the repair of a defect and/or restoration of a portion of a salivary gland duct.

D7983 closure of salivary fistula
Closure of an opening between a salivary duct and/or gland and the cutaneous surface, or an opening into the oral cavity through other than the normal anatomic pathway.

D7990 emergency tracheotomy
Formation of a tracheal opening usually below the cricoid cartilage to allow for respiratory exchange.

D7991 coronoidectomy
Removal of the coronoid process of the mandible.

D7995 synthetic graft – mandible or facial bones, by report
Includes allogenic material.

D7996 implant-mandible for augmentation purposes (excluding alveolar ridge), by report

D7997 appliance removal (not by dentist who placed appliance), includes removal of archbar

D7998 intraoral placement of a fixation device not in conjunction with a fracture
The placement of intermaxillary fixation appliance for documented medically accepted treatments not in association with fractures.

D7999 unspecified oral surgery procedure, by report
Used for procedure that is not adequately described by a code. Describe procedure.

  ● new procedure code ▲ revision to a nomenclature or descriptor

D8000-D8999 XI. Orthodontics

Dentition

Primary Dentition: Teeth developed and erupted first in order of time.

Transitional Dentition: The final phase of the transition from primary to adult teeth, in which the deciduous molars and canines are in the process of shedding and the permanent successors are emerging.

Adolescent Dentition: The dentition that is present after the normal loss of primary teeth and prior to cessation of growth that would affect orthodontic treatment.

Adult Dentition: The dentition that is present after the cessation of growth that would affect orthodontic treatment.

All of the following orthodontic treatment codes may be used more than once for the treatment of a particular patient depending on the particular circumstance. A patient may require more than one interceptive procedure or more than one limited procedure depending on their particular problem.

Limited Orthodontic Treatment

Orthodontic treatment with a limited objective, not necessarily involving the entire dentition. It may be directed at the only existing problem, or at only one aspect of a larger problem in which a decision is made to defer or forego more comprehensive therapy.

D8010 limited orthodontic treatment of the primary dentition

D8020 limited orthodontic treatment of the transitional dentition

D8030 limited orthodontic treatment of the adolescent dentition

D8040 limited orthodontic treatment of the adult dentition

Interceptive Orthodontic Treatment

Interceptive orthodontics is an extension of preventive orthodontics that may include localized tooth movement. Such treatment may occur in the primary or transitional dentition and may include such procedures as the redirection of ectopically erupting teeth, correction of dental crossbite or recovery of space loss where overall space is inadequate. When initiated during the incipient stages of a developing problem, interceptive orthodontics may reduce the severity of the malformation and mitigate its cause. Complicating factors such as skeletal disharmonies, overall space deficiency, or other conditions may require subsequent comprehensive therapy.

D8050 interceptive orthodontic treatment of the primary dentition

D8060 interceptive orthodontic treatment of the transitional dentition

Comprehensive Orthodontic Treatment

Comprehensive orthodontic care includes a coordinated diagnosis and treatment leading to the improvement of a patient's craniofacial dysfunction and/or dentofacial deformity which may include anatomical, functional and/or aesthetic relationships. Treatment may utilize fixed and/or removable orthodontic appliances and may also include functional and/or orthopedic appliances in growing and non-growing patients. Adjunctive procedures to facilitate care may be required. Comprehensive orthodontics may incorporate treatment phases focusing on specific objectives at various stages of dentofacial development.

D8070 comprehensive orthodontic treatment of the transitional dentition

D8080 comprehensive orthodontic treatment of the adolescent dentition

D8090 comprehensive orthodontic treatment of the adult dentition

● new procedure code   ▲ revision to a nomenclature or descriptor

Minor Treatment to Control Harmful Habits

D8210 **removable appliance therapy**
Removable indicates patient can remove; includes appliances for thumb sucking and tongue thrusting.

D8220 **fixed appliance therapy**
Fixed indicates patient cannot remove appliance; includes appliances for thumb sucking and tongue thrusting.

Other Orthodontic Services

D8660 **pre-orthodontic treatment examination to monitor growth and development**
Periodic observation of patient dentition, at intervals established by the dentist, to determine when orthodontic treatment should begin. Diagnostic procedures are documented separately.

D8670 **periodic orthodontic treatment visit**

D8680 **orthodontic retention (removal of appliances, construction and placement of retainer(s))**

D8681 **removable orthodontic retainer adjustment**

D8690 **orthodontic treatment (alternative billing to a contract fee)**
Services provided by dentist other than original treating dentist. A method of payment between the provider and responsible party for services that reflect an open-ended fee arrangement.

D8691 **repair of orthodontic appliance**
Does not include bracket and standard fixed orthodontic appliances. It does include functional appliances and palatal expanders.

D8692 **replacement of lost or broken retainer**

D8693 **re-cement or re-bond fixed retainer**

D8694 **repair of fixed retainers, includes reattachment**

• **D8695** **removal of fixed orthodontic appliances for reasons other than completion of treatment**

D8999   unspecified orthodontic procedure, by report
Used for procedure that is not adequately described by a code.
Describe procedure.

● new procedure code   ▲ revision to a nomenclature or descriptor

D9000-D9999 XII. Adjunctive General Services

Unclassified Treatment

D9110 palliative (emergency) treatment of dental pain – minor procedure
This is typically reported on a "per visit" basis for emergency treatment of dental pain.

D9120 fixed partial denture sectioning
Separation of one or more connections between abutments and/or pontics when some portion of a fixed prosthesis is to remain intact and serviceable following sectioning and extraction or other treatment. Includes all recontouring and polishing of retained portions.

Anesthesia

D9210 local anesthesia not in conjunction with operative or surgical procedures

D9211 regional block anesthesia

D9212 trigeminal division block anesthesia

D9215 local anesthesia in conjunction with operative or surgical procedures

D9219 evaluation for deep sedation or general anesthesia

• **D9222 deep sedation/general anesthesia – first 15 minutes**
Anesthesia time begins when the doctor administering the anesthetic agent initiates the appropriate anesthesia and non-invasive monitoring protocol and remains in continuous attendance of the patient. Anesthesia services are considered completed when the patient may be safely left under the observation of trained personnel and the doctor may safely leave the room to attend to other patients or duties.

The level of anesthesia is determined by the anesthesia provider's documentation of the anesthetic effects upon the central nervous system and not dependent upon the route of administration.

▲ **D9223** **deep sedation/general anesthesia – each subsequent 15 minute increment**

D9230 **inhalation of nitrous oxide/analgesia, anxiolysis**

• **D9239** **intravenous moderate (conscious) sedation/analgesia – first 15 minutes**
Anesthesia time begins when the doctor administering the anesthetic agent initiates the appropriate anesthesia and non-invasive monitoring protocol and remains in continuous attendance of the patient. Anesthesia services are considered completed when the patient may be safely left under the observation of trained personnel and the doctor may safely leave the room to attend to other patients or duties.

The level of anesthesia is determined by the anesthesia provider's documentation of the anesthetic effects upon the central nervous system and not dependent upon the route of administration.

▲ **D9243** **intravenous moderate (conscious) sedation/analgesia – each subsequent 15 minute increment**

D9248 **non-intravenous conscious sedation**
This includes non-IV minimal and moderate sedation.

A medically controlled state of depressed consciousness while maintaining the patient's airway, protective reflexes and the ability to respond to stimulation or verbal commands. It includes non-intravenous administration of sedative and/or analgesic agent(s) and appropriate monitoring.

The level of anesthesia is determined by the anesthesia provider's documentation of the anesthetic's effects upon the central nervous system and not dependent upon the route of administration.

Professional Consultation

D9310 **consultation – diagnostic service provided by dentist or physician other than requesting dentist or physician**
A patient encounter with a practitioner whose opinion or advice regarding evaluation and/or management of a specific problem; may be requested by another practitioner or appropriate source. The consultation includes an oral evaluation. The consulted practitioner may initiate diagnostic and/or therapeutic services.

D9311 **consultation with a medical health care professional**
Treating dentist consults with a medical health care professional concerning medical issues that may affect patient's planned dental treatment.

Professional Visits

D9410 **house/extended care facility call**
Includes visits to nursing homes, long-term care facilities, hospice sites, institutions, etc. Report in addition to reporting appropriate code numbers for actual services performed.

D9420 **hospital or ambulatory surgical center call**
Care provided outside the dentist's office to a patient who is in a hospital or ambulatory surgical center. Services delivered to the patient on the date of service are documented separately using the applicable procedure codes.

D9430 **office visit for observation (during regularly scheduled hours) – no other services performed**

D9440 **office visit – after regularly scheduled hours**

D9450 **case presentation, detailed and extensive treatment planning**
Established patient. Not performed on same day as evaluation.

Drugs

D9610 therapeutic parenteral drug, single administration
Includes single administration of antibiotics, steroids, anti-inflammatory drugs, or other therapeutic medications. This code should not be used to report administration of sedative, anesthetic or reversal agents.

D9612 therapeutic parenteral drugs, two or more administrations, different medications
Includes multiple administrations of antibiotics, steroids, anti-inflammatory drugs or other therapeutic medications. This code should not be used to report administration of sedatives, anesthetic or reversal agents.

This code should be reported when two or more different medications are necessary and should not be reported in addition to code D9610 on the same date.

D9630 drugs or medicaments dispensed in the office for home use
Includes, but is not limited to oral antibiotics, oral analgesics, and topical fluoride; does not include writing prescriptions.

Miscellaneous Services

D9910 application of desensitizing medicament
Includes in-office treatment for root sensitivity. Typically reported on a "per visit" basis for application of topical fluoride. This code is not to be used for bases, liners or adhesives used under restorations.

D9911 application of desensitizing resin for cervical and/or root surface, per tooth
Typically reported on a "per tooth" basis for application of adhesive resins. This code is not to be used for bases, liners, or adhesives used under restorations.

D9920 behavior management, by report
May be reported in addition to treatment provided. Should be reported in 15-minute increments.

D9930 treatment of complications (post-surgical) – unusual circumstances, by report
For example, treatment of a dry socket following extraction or removal of bony sequestrum.

D9932 **cleaning and inspection of removable complete denture, maxillary**
This procedure does not include any adjustments.

D9933 **cleaning and inspection of removable complete denture, mandibular**
This procedure does not include any adjustments.

D9934 **cleaning and inspection of removable partial denture, maxillary**
This procedure does not include any adjustments.

D9935 **cleaning and inspection of removable partial denture, mandibular**
This procedure does not include any adjustments.

D9940 **occlusal guard, by report**
Removable dental appliances, which are designed to minimize the effects of bruxism (grinding) and other occlusal factors.

D9941 **fabrication of athletic mouthguard**

D9942 **repair and/or reline of occlusal guard**

D9943 **occlusal guard adjustment**

D9950 **occlusion analysis – mounted case**
Includes, but is not limited to, facebow, interocclusal records tracings, and diagnostic wax-up; for diagnostic casts, see D0470.

D9951 **occlusal adjustment – limited**
May also be known as equilibration; reshaping the occlusal surfaces of teeth to create harmonious contact relationships between the maxillary and mandibular teeth. Presently includes discing/odontoplasty/enamoplasty. Typically reported on a "per visit" basis. This should not be reported when the procedure only involves bite adjustment in the routine post-delivery care for a direct/indirect restoration or fixed/removable prosthodontics.

D9952 occlusal adjustment – complete
Occlusal adjustment may require several appointments of varying length, and sedation may be necessary to attain adequate relaxation of the musculature. Study casts mounted on an articulating instrument may be utilized for analysis of occlusal disharmony. It is designed to achieve functional relationships and masticatory efficiency in conjunction with restorative treatment, orthodontics, orthognathic surgery, or jaw trauma when indicated. Occlusal adjustment enhances the healing potential of tissues affected by the lesions of occlusal trauma.

D9970 enamel microabrasion
The removal of discolored surface enamel defects resulting from altered mineralization or decalcification of the superficial enamel layer. Submit per treatment visit.

D9971 odontoplasty 1-2 teeth; includes removal of enamel projections

D9972 external bleaching – per arch – performed in office

D9973 external bleaching – per tooth

D9974 internal bleaching – per tooth

D9975 external bleaching for home application, per arch; includes materials and fabrication of custom trays

Non-clinical procedures

D9985 sales tax

D9986 missed appointment

D9987 cancelled appointment

D9991 dental case management – addressing appointment compliance barriers
Individualized efforts to assist a patient to maintain scheduled appointments by solving transportation challenges or other barriers.

● new procedure code   ▲ revision to a nomenclature or descriptor

D9992 **dental case management – care coordination**
Assisting in a patient's decisions regarding the coordination of oral health care services across multiple providers, provider types, specialty areas of treatment, health care settings, health care organizations and payment systems. This is the additional time and resources expended to provide experience or expertise beyond that possessed by the patient.

D9993 **dental case management – motivational interviewing**
Patient-centered, personalized counseling using methods such as Motivational Interviewing (MI) to identify and modify behaviors interfering with positive oral health outcomes. This is a separate service from traditional nutritional or tobacco counseling.

D9994 **dental case management – patient education to improve oral health literacy**
Individual, customized communication of information to assist the patient in making appropriate health decisions designed to improve oral health literacy, explained in a manner acknowledging economic circumstances and different cultural beliefs, values, attitudes, traditions and language preferences, and adopting information and services to these differences, which requires the expenditure of time and resources beyond that of an oral evaluation or case presentation.

• **D9995** **teledentistry – synchronous; real-time encounter**
Reported in addition to other procedures (e.g., diagnostic) delivered to the patient on the date of service.

• **D9996** **teledentistry – asynchronous; information stored and forwarded to dentist for subsequent review**
Reported in addition to other procedures (e.g., diagnostic) delivered to the patient on the date of service.

D9999 **unspecified adjunctive procedure, by report**
Used for procedure that is not adequately described by a code. Describe procedure.

PRACTICAL
GUIDE
SERIES

2

Changes to the CDT Code

ADA American Dental Association®
America's leading advocate for oral health

Changes to the CDT Code

This version of the CDT Code is effective January 1, 2018 through December 31, 2018. All changes are illustrated in this section, with added text <u>underlined in blue ink</u> and deleted text ~~stricken through in red ink~~. There are:

- 18 Additions

- 16 Revisions

- 3 Deletions

- 0 Editorial (e.g., syntax; spelling) actions that clarify without changing the CDT Code entry's purpose or scope

As noted in the preface, the CDT Code is divided into twelve Categories of Service <u>only</u> for the purpose of organization. Each category begins at the top of a right-hand page in this section.

Classification of Materials

Additions
None

Revisions
None

Deletions
None

Editorial
None

D0100-D0999 I. Diagnostic

Additions
One (1) CDT Code

D0411 **HbA1c in-office point of service testing**

Revisions
None

Deletions
None

Editorial
None

D1000-D1999 II. Preventive

Additions
None

Revisions
Two (2) CDT Codes

D1354 **interim caries arresting medicament application – per tooth**
Conservative treatment of an active, non-symptomatic carious lesion by topical application of a caries arresting or inhibiting medicament and without mechanical removal of sound tooth structure.

D1555 **removal of fixed space maintainer**
Procedure ~~delivered~~ performed by dentist or practice that ~~who~~ did not originally place the appliance~~, or by the practice where the appliance was originally delivered to the patient~~.

Deletions
None

Editorial
None

D2000–D2999   III. Restorative

Additions
None

Revisions
One (1) CDT Code

D2740   crown – porcelain/ceramic ~~substrate~~

Deletions
None

Editorial
None

D3000-D3999   IV. Endodontics

Additions
None

Revisions
Five (5) CDT Codes

D3320   **endodontic therapy, <u>premolar</u> ~~bicuspid~~ tooth (excluding final restoration)**

D3330   **endodontic therapy, molar <u>tooth</u> (excluding final restoration)**

D3347   **retreatment of previous root canal therapy – ~~bicuspid~~ <u>premolar</u>**

D3421   **apicoectomy – ~~bicuspid~~ <u>premolar</u> (first root)**
For surgery on one root of a bicuspid premolar. Does not include placement of retrograde filling material. If more than one root is treated, see D3426.

D3426   **apicoectomy – (each additional root)**
Typically used for ~~bicuspids~~ <u>premolar</u> and molar surgeries when more than one root is treated during the same procedure. This does not include retrograde filling material placement.

Deletions
None

Editorial
None

D4000-D4999   V. Periodontics

Additions
None

Revisions
Three (3) CDT Codes

D4230   **anatomical crown exposure – four or more contiguous teeth** <u>**or bounded tooth spaces**</u> **per quadrant**
This procedure is utilized in an otherwise periodontally healthy area to remove enlarged gingival tissue and supporting bone (ostectomy) to provide anatomically correct gingival relationship.

D4231   **anatomical crown exposure – one to three teeth** <u>**or bounded tooth spaces**</u> **per quadrant**
This procedure is utilized in an otherwise periodontally healthy area to remove enlarged gingival tissue and supporting bone (ostectomy) to provide an anatomically correct gingival relationship.

D4355   **full mouth debridement to enable a comprehensive oral evaluation and diagnosis** <u>**on a subsequent visit**</u>
~~The gross~~ <u>Full mouth debridement involves the preliminary</u> removal of plaque and calculus that interferes with the ability of the dentist to perform a comprehensive oral evaluation. ~~This preliminary procedure does not preclude the need for additional procedures.~~ <u>Not to be completed on the same day as D0150, D0160, or D0180.</u>

Deletions
None

Editorial
None

D5000-D5899   VI. Prosthodontics (removable)

Additions
Six (6) CDT Codes

D5511   repair broken complete denture base, mandibular

D5512   repair broken complete denture base, maxillary

D5611   repair resin partial denture base, mandibular

D5612   repair resin partial denture base, maxillary

D5621   repair cast partial framework, mandibular

D5622   repair cast partial framework, maxillary

Revisions
None

Deletions
Three (3) CDT Codes

D5510   repair broken complete denture base

D5610   repair resin denture base

D5620   repair cast framework

Editorial
None

D5900-D5999 VII. Maxillofacial Prosthetics

Additions
None

Revisions
None

Deletions
None

Editorial
None

D6000–D6199 VIII. Implant Services

Additions
Three (3) CDT Codes

D6096 **remove broken implant retaining screw**

D6118 **implant/abutment supported interim fixed denture for edentulous arch – mandibular**
Used when a period of healing is necessary prior to fabrication and placement of a permanent prosthetic.

D6119 **implant/abutment supported interim fixed denture for edentulous arch – maxillary**
Used when a period of healing is necessary prior to fabrication and placement of a permanent prosthetic

Revisions
One (1) CDT Code

D6081 **scaling and debridement in the pres ence of inflammation or mucositis of a single implant, including cleaning of the implant surfaces, without flap entry and closure**
This procedure is not performed in conjunction with D1110, ~~or~~ D4910, or D4346.

Deletions
None

Editorial
None

D6200-D6999   IX. Prosthodontics, fixed

Additions
None

Revisions
None

Deletions
None

Editorial
None

D7000-D7999   X. Oral and Maxillofacial Surgery

Additions
Three (3) CDT Codes

D7296 **corticotomy – one to three teeth or tooth spaces, per quadrant**
This procedure involves creating multiple cuts, perforations, or removal of cortical, alveolar or basal bone of the jaw for the purpose of facilitating orthodontic repositioning of the dentition. This procedure includes flap entry and closure. Graft material and membrane, if used, should be reported separately.

D7297 **corticotomy – four or more teeth or tooth spaces, per quadrant**
This procedure involves creating multiple cuts, perforations, or removal of cortical, alveolar or basal bone of the jaw for the purpose of facilitating orthodontic repositioning of the dentition. This procedure includes flap entry and closure. Graft material and membrane, if used, should be reported separately.

D7979 **non – surgical sialolithotomy**
A sialolith is removed from the gland or ductal portion of the gland without surgical incision into the gland or the duct of the gland; for example via manual manipulation, ductal dilation, or any other non-surgical method.

Revisions
Two (2) CDT Codes

D7111 **extraction, coronal remnants – primary** ~~deciduous~~ **tooth**
Removal of soft tissue – retained coronal remnants.

D7980 **surgical sialolithotomy**
Procedure by which a stone within a salivary gland or its duct is removed, either intraorally or extraorally.

Deletions
None

Editorial

None

D8000-D8999   XI. Orthodontics

Additions
One (1) CDT Code

D8695   **removal of fixed orthodontic appliances for reasons other than completion of treatment**

Revisions
None

Deletions
None

Editorial
None

D9000-D9999 XII. Adjunctive General Services

Additions
Five (5) CDT Codes

D9222 **deep sedation/general anesthesia – first 15 minutes**
Anesthesia time begins when the doctor administering the anesthetic agent initiates the appropriate anesthesia and non-invasive monitoring protocol and remains in continuous attendance of the patient. Anesthesia services are considered completed when the patient may be safely left under the observation of trained personnel and the doctor may safely leave the room to attend to other patients or duties.

The level of anesthesia is determined by the anesthesia provider's documentation of the anesthetic effects upon the central nervous system and not dependent upon the route of administration.

D9239 **intravenous moderate (conscious) sedation/analgesia – first 15 minutes**
Anesthesia time begins when the doctor administering the anesthetic agent initiates the appropriate anesthesia and non-invasive monitoring protocol and remains in continuous attendance of the patient. Anesthesia services are considered completed when the patient may be safely left under the observation of trained personnel and the doctor may safely leave the room to attend to other patients or duties.

The level of anesthesia is determined by the anesthesia provider's documentation of the anesthetic effects upon the central nervous system and not dependent upon the route of administration.

D9995 **teledentistry – synchronous; real-time encounter**
Reported in addition to other procedures (e.g., diagnostic) delivered to the patient on the date of service.

D9996 **teledentistry – asynchronous; information stored and forwarded to dentist for subsequent review**
Reported in addition to other procedures (e.g., diagnostic) delivered to the patient on the date of service.

Revisions
Two (2) CDT Codes

D9223 deep sedation/general anesthesia – each <u>subsequent</u> 15 minute increment

~~Anesthesia time begins when the doctor administering the anesthetic agent initiates the appropriate anesthesia and non-invasive monitoring protocol and remains in continuous attendance of the patient. Anesthesia services are considered completed when the patient may be safely left under the observation of trained personnel and the doctor may safely leave the room to attend to other patients or duties.~~

~~The level of anesthesia is determined by the anesthesia provider's documentation of the anesthetics effects upon the central nervous system and not dependent upon the route of administration.~~

D9243 intravenous moderate (conscious) sedation/analgesia – each <u>subsequent</u> 15 minute increment

~~Anesthesia time begins when the doctor administering the anesthetic agent initiates the appropriate anesthesia and non-invasive monitoring protocol and remains in continuous attendance of the patient. Anesthesia services are considered completed when the patient may be safely left under the observation of trained personnel and the doctor may safely leave the room to attend to other patients or duties.~~

~~The level of anesthesia is determined by the anesthesia provider's documentation of the anesthetics effects upon the central nervous system and not dependent upon the route of administration.~~

Deletions
None

Editorial
None

PRACTICAL
GUIDE
SERIES

3

Alphabetic Index to
the CDT Code

ADA American Dental Association®
America's leading advocate for oral health

Alphabetic Index to the CDT Code

Term	Code(s)	Page(s)
A		
A1c testing	D0411	10
Abscess, incision and drainage, all types	D7510, D7511, D7520, D7521	74
Abutments	Also see **Retainers**	
for implants	D6051, D6056, D6057	59
Accession of tissue	D0472 – D0474	12
Acid etch; part of resin procedure	No separate code	
Adhesives, bonding agents (resin and and amalgam bonding agents); part of restorative procedure	No separate code	
Adjunctive General Services (Category of Service)	D9000 – D9999	87-93
Adjunctive pre-diagnostic test	D0431	11
Adjust		
prosthetic appliance	D5992	47
orthodontic retainer	D8681	85
Allograft, soft tissue	D4275, D7955	37, 81
Alveoloplasty	D7310, D7311, D7320, D7321	72
Alveolus, fracture	D7670, D7671, D7770, D7771	75-76
Amalgam restorations	D2140 – D2161	20
Amalgam and resin bonding agents (part of restorative procedure)	No separate code	
Analgesia		
inhalation of nitrous oxide	D9230	88
non-intravenous conscious sedation	D9248	88

Term	Code(s)	Page(s)
Anchorage device, temporary		
requiring flap	D7293	71
without flap	D7294	71
screw retained plate requiring flap	D7292	71
Anesthesia		
evaluation for...general	D9219	87
general	D9222, D9223	87-88
local	D9210, D9215	87
regional	D9211	87
trigeminal division block	D9212	87
Ankyloglossia	See **frenectomy/frenotomy (frenulectomy)**	
Apexification/recalcification	D3351 – D3353	29-30
Apexogenesis	D3222	28
Apically positioned flap	D4245	35
Apicoectomy	D3410 – D3426	30-31
Appliance removal (not by dentist who placed)	D7997	82
Arthrocentesis	D7870	78
Appointment		
cancelled	D9987	92
missed	D9986	92
Arthroplasty	D7865	77
Arthroscopy	D7872 – D7877	78
Arthrotomy	D7860	77

Term	Code(s)	Page(s)
Assessment of a patient	D0191	7
Athletic mouthguard	D9941	91
Autologous blood concentrate (collection and application)	D7921	79

B

Bacteriologic studies	D0415	10
Behavior management	D9920	90
Biologic materials	D4265	36
in conjunction with periradicular surgery	D3431	31
Biopsy		
brush	D7288	71
hard tissue	D7285	71
soft tissue	D7286	71
Bitewing radiographs	D0270 – D0277	8
Bleaching		
external – per arch	D9972	92
external – per tooth	D9973	92
external – for home application	D9975	92
internal – per tooth	D9974	92
Bone fragment (post-surgical removal)	D9930	90
Bone, harvest of	D7295	71
Bone tissue, excision	D7471 – D7490	74
Bonding agents; adhesives (resin and amalgam bonding agents)	No separate code – part of restorative procedure	
Bridge	See **Fixed Partial Dentures**	

Term	Code(s)	Page(s)
Composite resin	See Resin-based composite (direct and indirect)	
Comprehensive orthodontics	D8070 – D8090	84
Condylectomy	D7840	77
Cone Beam – CT		
image capture and interpretation	D0364 – D0368	9
image capture only	D0380 – D0384	9
interpretation and report only	D0391	10
post processing image or image sets	D0393 – D0395	10
Connector bar		
dental implant supported	D6055	59
fixed partial denture	D6920	68
Conscious sedation	D9239, D9243, D9248	88
Consultation		
patient referred by another practitioner	D9310	89
dentist with other health care professional	D9311	89
Coping	D2975	25
Core buildup	D2950	24
Corticotomy	D7296, D7297	72
Coronectomy	D7251	70
Coronoidectomy	D7991	82
Counseling		
nutritional	D1310	15
tobacco	D1320	15
oral hygiene	D1330	15

Term	Code(s)	Page(s)
Crevicular antimicrobial agents	D4381	40
Crown		
abutment (on implant) supported	D6058 – D6064, D6094	60-61
implant supported	D6065 – D6067	61
individual restorations (indirect)	D2710 – D2799	22-23
prefabricated	D2929 – D2934	23-24
provisional		
single restoration	D2799	23
implant	D6085	63
re-cement	D2920	23
repair	D2980	25
resin-based composite, anterior, direct	D2390	20
under existing removable partial	D2971	25
zirconia / zirconium	D2740	22
Crown exposure	D4230, D4231	34
Crown lengthening, hard tissue	D4249	35
Crown repair	D2980	25
Cryosurgery	D7465	73
Culture and sensitivity		
collection of microorganisms	D0415	10
laboratory processing of specimen	D0414	10
Culture, viral	D0416	10
Curettage		

Term	Code(s)	Page(s)
open flap	D4240, D4241	34
without flap	D4341, D4342	39
Cysts, removal of	D7410 – D7465	73
Cytologic smears	D0480	12
Cytology sample collection	D7287	71

D

Debridement		
endodontic	D3221	27
full mouth	D4355	39
single implant	D6081	63
peri-implant	D6101 – D6102	58
Dental Case Management		
addressing appointment compliance	D9991	92
care coordination	D9992	93
motivational interviewing	D9993	93
patient education	D9994	93
Dentures (removable)		
adjustments	D5410 – D5422	42
complete	D5110 – D5120	41
immediate, complete	D5130, D5140	41
implant/abutment supported, complete	D6110, D6111	59
implant/abutment supported, partial	D6112, D6113	59
modification of removable prosthesis following implant surgery	D5875	45

Term	Code(s)	Page(s)
overdenture	D5863 – D5866	45
partial	D5211 – D5281	41-42
precision attachment	D5862	45
rebase	D5710 – D5721	43
reline	D5730 – D5761	44
repairs, complete and partial	D5511, D5512, D5520, D5611, D5612, D5621, D5622, D5671	43
temporary/interim	D5810 – D5821	44
Dentures (fixed)		
implant/abutment supported, full	D6114, D6115	59
implant/abutment supported, partial	D6116, D6117	59-60
implant/abutment supported, interim	D6118, D6119	60
Desensitizing medicament	D9910	90
Desensitizing resin	D9911	90
Destruction of lesion	D7465	73
Diabetes testing (A1c)	D0411	10
Diagnostic (Category of Service)	D0100 – D0999	5-13
Diagnostic casts	D0470	11
Diagnostic imaging		
image capture and interpretation	D0210 – D0371	7-9
image capture only	D0380 – D0386	9-10
interpretation and report only	D0391	10
post processing image or image sets	D0393 – D0395	10
Disc repair (TMJ)	D7852	77

Term	Code(s)	Page(s)
Dietary planning (nutritional counseling)	D1310	15
Distal shoe space maintainer	D1575	17
Dressing change, periodontal, unscheduled	D4920	40
Drugs		
therapeutic parenteral, single administration	D9610	90
therapeutic parental, two or more administrations	D9612	90
drugs or medicaments	D9630	90
Dry socket/localized osteitis	D9930	90

E

Term	Code(s)	Page(s)
Emergency treatment	D0140, D9110	5, 87
Enamel microabrasion	D9970	92
Enameloplasty	D9971	92
Endodontics (Category of Service)	D3000 – D3999	27-32
Endodontic endosseous implant	D3460	31
Equilibration (occlusal adjustment)	D9951, D9952	91-92
Eruption of teeth		
mobilization, surgical	D7282	70
placement of device to aid eruption	D7283	70
Evaluations		
periodic – established patient	D0120	5
limited – problem focused	D0140	5
for patient under 3 years & counseling with primary caregiver	D0145	5

Term	Code(s)	Page(s)
comprehensive – new or established patient	D0150	6
detailed and extensive – problem focused, by report	D0160	6
re-evaluation – limited	D0170	6
re-evaluation – post operative office visit	D0171	7
comprehensive periodontal – new or established patient	D0180	7
pre-orthodontic (examination)	D8660	85
Excision		
benign lesion	D7410 – D7412	73
malignant lesion/tumor	D7413 – D7415, D7440, D7441	73
Exfoliative cytological smear	D0480	12
Exostosis (tuberosity); removal of		
lateral exostosis	D7471	74
osseous tuberosity	D7485	74
surgical reduction of fibrous tuberosity	D7972	81
torus palatinus	D7472	74
torus mandibularis	D7473	74
Extraoral Images (radiographic)	D0250, D0251	8
Extractions	D7111, D7140, D7210-D7250	69-70

F

Facial Bone Survey	D0250	8
Fiberotomy, transseptal	D7291	71

Term	Code(s)	Page(s)
Fibroma	D7410, D7411	73
Fissurotomy	see **Odontoplasty**	
Fistula		
oroantral	D7260	70
salivary	D7983	82
Fixation device, not in conjunction with fracture	D7998	82
Fixed partial dentures (bridges)		
pontics	D6205 – D6253	65
re-cementation	D6930	68
repair	D6980	68
retainers		
crowns	D6710 – D6794	67
implant/abutment supported	D6068 – D6077, D6194	61-62
inlay/onlay	D6600 – D6634	66
Maryland Bridge	D6545, D6548, D6549	66
pediatric	D6985	68
sectioning	D9120	87
Flaps		
apically positioned	D4245	35
gingival	D4240, D4241	34
Flexible base partial denture	D5225, D5226	42
"Flipper", interim/transitional removable prosthesis (aka "stayplate")	D5820, D5821	44
Fluoride		

Term	Code(s)	Page(s)
Frenectomy/frenotomy (frenulectomy)	D7960	81
Frenuloplasty	D7963	81
Full mouth series	D0210	7

G

Genetic testing		
sample collection	D0422	11
specimen analysis	D0423	11
Gingiva, pericoronal, removal of	D7971	81
Gingival flap	D4240, D4241	34
Gingival Irrigation	D4921	40
Gingivectomy/gingivoplasty	D4210, D4211, D4212	33-34
Glass ionomers (resin restorations)	D2330 – D2394	20-21
Gold foil	D2410 – D2430	21
Graft		
bone replacement	D4263, D4264, D6103, D6104, D7953	36, 58, 80
combined connective tissue and double pedicle	D4276	38
free soft tissue	D4277 – D4278	38
maxillofacial soft/hard tissue	D7955	81
osseous, osteoperiosteal, or cartilage	D7950	80
pedicle soft tissue	D4270	37
periradicular	D3428, D3429	31
sinus augmentation	D7951	80
skin	D7920	79

Term	Code(s)	Page(s)
soft tissue	D4270 – D4273	37
connective tissue		
autogenous	D4273, D4283	37
non-autogenous	D4275, D4285	37–38
synthetic	D7955	81
Guided tissue regeneration	D4266, D4267	36–37
in conjunction with periradicular surgery	D3432	31

H

Term	Code(s)	Page(s)
Harvest of bone	D7295	71
Hemisection	D3920	32
Hospital call (hospital or ambulatory surgicenter visit)	D9420	89
House call (nursing home visit)	D9410	89
Hyperplastic tissue removal	D7970	81

I

Term	Code(s)	Page(s)
Images, oral/facial	D0350	8
Immediate denture		
complete	D5130, D5140	41
partial	D5221 – D5224	41–42
Impacted tooth, removal of	D7220 – D7241	69
Implant		
abutments	D6056, D6057, D6051	59
chin	D7995	82
endodontic	D3460	31

Term	Code(s)	Page(s)
endosteal/endosseous	D6010	57
eposteal/subperiosteal	D6040	57
interim implant	D6012	57
maintenance	D6080	63
mandible	D7996	82
mini	D6013	57
modification of removable prosthesis	D5875	45
other implant services	D6080 – D6199	63-64
peri-implant defect	D6103	58
radiographic/surgical implant index	D6190	57
re-cement	D6092, D6093	63
removal	D6100	58
repair	D6090, D6091, D6095	63
retaining screw (broken) removal	D6096	63
scaling and debridement	D6081	63
second stage surgery	D6011	57
transosteal/transosseous	D6050	58
Implant Services (Category of Service)	D6000 – D6199	57-64
Implantation (of tooth)	See **Re-implantation**	
Incision and drainage	D7510, D7511, D7520, D7521	74
Inlay		
fixed partial denture retainer		
metallic	D6602 – D6607, D6624	66
porcelain/ceramic	D6600 – D6601	66

Term	Code(s)	Page(s)
metallic	D2510 – D2530	21
porcelain/ceramic	D2610 – D2630	21
re-cement	D2910	23
resin-based composite	D2650 – D2652	22
Intentional re-implantation	D3470	31
Interceptive orthodontics	D8050, D8060	84
Interim abutment	D6051	59
Interim complete denture	D5810, D5811	44
Interim partial denture	D5820, D5821	44
Internal root repair	D3333	29
Interpretation of diagnostic image (different practitioner)	D0391	10
Intravenous moderate (conscious) sedation/analgesia	D9239, D9243	88
Irrigation (gingival)	D4921	40

J

Joint reconstruction	D7858	77

K

No "K" terms

L

Labial veneer	D2960, D2961, D2962	25
Laser	No separate code – part of dental procedure code that appropriately describes the service provided	
Lateral exostosis	D7471	74

Term	Code(s)	Page(s)
LeFort I	D7946, D7947	80
LeFort II; LeFort III	D7948, D7949	80
Lesions, surgical excision		
intra-osseous lesions	D7440 – D7461	73-74
soft tissue	D7410 – D7415, D7465	73
Limited orthodontic treatment	D8010 – D8040	83
Localized osteitis/dry socket	D9930	90

M

Maintenance and cleaning of prosthesis	D5993	47
Malar bone, repair of fracture	D7650, D7660, D7750, D7760	75-76
Malocclusion, correction of	D8000 – D8999	83-86
Mandible, fracture of	D7630 – D7640, D7730 – D7740	75-76
Maryland Bridge (resin bonded fixed prosthesis)		
retainer/abutment	D6545, D6548, D6549	66
pontic	D6210 – D6252	65
Maxilla, repair of fracture	D7610 – D7620, D7710 D7720	75-76
Maxillofacial defect	D7955	81
Maxillofacial MRI		
capture and interpretation	D0369	9
image capture (only)	D0385	10
Maxillofacial Prosthetics (Category of Service)	D5900 - D5999	47-56
adjust prosthetic appliance	D5992	47

Term	Code(s)	Page(s)
maintenance and cleaning of prosthesis	D5993	47
Maxillofacial ultrasound		
capture and interpretation	D0370	9
image capture (only)	D0386	10
Mesial/distal wedge	D4274	38
Metals, classification of		4
Microabrasion, enamel	D9970	92
Microorganisms, culture and sensitivity	D0415	10
Minimal (mild) sedation	D9248	88
Missed appointment	D9986	92
Moderate sedation	D9239, D9243, D9248	88
Moulage, facial	D5911, D5912	48
Mouthguard, athletic	D9941	91
Mucosal abnormalities, pre–diagnostic test	D0431	11
Myotomy	D7856	77

N

Term	Code(s)	Page(s)
Neoplasms, removal of	D7410 – D7465	73
Nightguard	D9940	91
Nitrous oxide, analgesia	D9230	88
Non-intravenous moderate (conscious) sedation	D9248	88
Non-odontogenic cyst	D7460, D7461	74
Nursing home, (house/extended care facility visit)	D9410	89

Term	Code(s)	Page(s)
Oral & Maxillofacial Surgery (Category of Service)	D7000 – D7999	69-82
Oral hygiene instructions	D1330	15
Oral pathology		
accession of tissue	D0472 – D0474; D0480, D0486	12
consultation, slides	D0484, D0485	13
cytology	D0480	12
decalcification procedure	D0475	12
electron microscopy	D0481	13
immunofluorescence		
direct	D0482	13
indirect	D0483	13
immunohistochemical stains	D0478	13
other oral pathology procedures	D0502	13
special stains	D0476, D0477	12-13
tissue hybridization	D0479	13
Orthodontics (Category of Service)	D8000 – D8999	83-86
Orthodontic treatment (not by the original treating dentist)	D8690	85
Orthotic appliance	D7880	78
Osseous surgery/graft	D4260 – D4264	35-36
Ostectomy, partial	D7550	75
Osteitis, localized; dry socket	D9930	90
Osteoplasty	D7940	79
Osteotomy	D7941 – D7945	79

Term	Code(s)	Page(s)
Provisional		
single crown	D2799	23
pontic (FPD)	D6253	65
implant crown	D6085	63
retainer crown (FPD)	D6793	67
Pulp cap	D3110, D3120	27
Pulp vitality tests	D0460	11
Pulpal debridement	D3221	27
Pupal regeneration	D3355 – D3357	30
Pulpal therapy, primary teeth	D3230, D3240	28
Pulpotomy		
therapeutic (excluding final restoration)	D3220	27
partial for apexogenesis	D3222	28
Q		
No "Q" terms.		
R		
Radiation		
carrier	D5983	56
cone locator	D5985	53
shield	D5984	54
Radiographic/surgical implant index	D6190	57
Radiographs		
image capture and interpretation	D0210 – D0340	7-8

Term	Code(s)	Page(s)
interpretation and report only	D0391	10
Reattach tooth fragment	D2921	23
Recalcification/apexification	D3351 – D3353	29-30
Re-cement		
bridge	D6930	68
crown	D2920	23
fixed retainers	D8693	85
implant fixed partial denture	D6093	63
implant crown	D6092	63
inlay	D2910	23
onlay	D2910	23
post and core	D2915	23
space maintainer	D1550	16
veneer	D2910	23
Re-implantation		
intentional	D3470	31
accidentally evulsed or displaced	D7270	70
Removable partial denture	See **Partial Dentures**	
Repair		
complete removable denture	D5511, D5512, D5520	43
crown	D2980	25
fixed partial denture	D6980	68
implant precision or semi-precision attachment	D6091	63
inlay	D2981	25

Term	Code(s)	Page(s)
occlusal guard	D9942	91
onlay	D2982	25
orthodontic appliance	D8691	85
orthodontic fixed retainer	D8693, D8694	85
precision or semi-precision attachment	D5867, D6052	45, 59
removable partial dentures	D5611, D5612, D5621, D5622 – D5671	43
sealant	D1353	16
veneer	D2983	25
Resin, definition of		4
Resin-based composite, direct		
anterior	D2330 – D2335	20
crown	D2390	20
posterior	D2391 – D2394	20-21
veneers	D2960	25
Resin-based composite, indirect		
crown	D2710	22
fixed partial denture abutment	D6710	67
inlay/onlay	D2650 – D2664	22
pontic	D6205	65
¾ crown	D2712	22
veneers	D2961	25
Restorations		
amalgam	D2140 – D2161	20

Term	Code(s)	Page(s)
gold foil	D2410 – D2430	21
inlay/onlay	D2510 – D2664	21-22
	D6600 – D6634	66
interim therapeutic	D2941	24
resin-based composite	D2330 – D2394	20-21
resin infiltration	D2990	23
preventive resin	D1352	16
protective	D2940	24
Restorative (Category of Service)	D2000 – D2999	19-25
Restorative foundation for indirect restoration	D2949	24
Retainers		
fixed partial denture		
resin bonded (aka "Maryland Bridge")	D6545, D6548, D6549	66
inlays/onlays	D6600 – D6634	66
crowns	D6710 – D6794	67
implant abutment supported	D6068 – D6074, D6194	61-62
implant supported	D6075 – D6077	62
orthodontic	D8680, D8691, D8692	85
Retreatment, endodontic	D3346 – D3348	29
Retrograde filling	D3430	31
Revision, periodontal surgery	D4268	37
Ridge augmentation (grafting)	D7950	80
Root		
planing	D4341	39

Term	Code(s)	Page(s)
Section of fixed partial denture	D9120	87
Sedation		
evaluation for deep/general	D9219	87
deep	D9222, D9223	87-88
intravenous, moderate (conscious)	D9239, D9243	88
non-intravenous conscious		
minimal (mild)	D9248	88
moderate	D9248	88
Sedative filling	See **Protective Restoration**	
Semi-precision attachment abutment	D6052	59
Sequestrectomy	D7550	75
Sialodochoplasty	D7982	82
Sialoendoscopy capture and interpretation	D0371	9
Sialography	D0310	8
Sialolithotomy		
non-surgical	D7979	81
surgical	D7980	81
Sinus augmentation		
via lateral open approach	D7951	80
via vertical approach	D7952	80
Sinus perforation, closure	D7261	70
Sinusotomy	D7560	75
Skin graft	D7920	79

Term	Code(s)	Page(s)
Sleep apnea appliance	D5999	56
Space maintainer	D1510 – D1575	16-17
distal shoe	D1575	17
re-cement	D1550	16
removal (by dentist who did not place appliance)	D1555	16
Speech aid		
adult	D5953	54
pediatric	D5952	54
Splinting		
commissure	D5987	47
provisional	D4320, D4321	38
surgical	D5988	55
Stainless steel crown	D2930, D2931, D2933, D2934	23-24
Stayplate (aka "flipper")	D5820, D5821	44
Stent	D5982	55
Stress breaker	D6940	68
Supra crestal fiberotomy	D7291	71
Surgical/ambulatory center	D9420	89
Suturing		
simple	D7910	79
complicated	D7911, D7912	79
Synovectomy	D7854	77

Term	Code(s)	Page(s)
T		
Teledentistry		
Synchronous; real time encounter	D9995	93
Asynchronous ("store and forward")	D9996	93
Temporomandibular joint (TMJ)		
manipulation	D7830	77
radiographs	D0320, D0321	8
reduction	D7810 – D7820	77
surgical discectomy	D7850	77
treatment	D7810 – D7899	77-78
Thumb sucking appliance	D8210, D8220	85
Tissue conditioning	D5850, D5851	45
Tissue, excision of hyperplastic	D7970	81
Titanium		
crown, FPD retainer	D6794	67
crown, single unit	D2794	23
implant abutment supported	D6094	61
implant abutment supported for FPD	D6194	62
implant supported	D6065	61
implant supported for FPD	D6067	61
inlay, FPD retainer	D6624	66
onlay, FPD retainer	D6634	66
pontic	D6214	65

Term	Code(s)	Page(s)
Tuberosity		
fibrous	D7972	81
osseous (reduction, surgical)	D7485	74
Tumors, (removal of)	D7440 – D7465	73

U

Term	Code(s)	Page(s)
Un-erupted tooth, access	D7280	70
Unilateral removable partial denture	D5281	42

V

Term	Code(s)	Page(s)
Veneers	D2960 – D2962	25
Vertical bitewings	D0277	8
Vestibuloplasty	D7340, D7350	73
Viral culture	D0416	10

W

Term	Code(s)	Page(s)
Wax-up (diagnostic)	D9950	91
Wedge - mesial/distal	D4274	38
Whitening	See **Bleaching**	
Wounds, treatment of	D7910 – D7912	79

X

Term	Code(s)	Page(s)
X-rays	See **Diagnostic Imaging**	

Y

No "Y" terms.

Term	Code(s)	Page(s)
Z		
Zirconia / Zirconium	Use applicable "porcelain/ceramic" prosthesis code from Restorative, Prosthodontic or Implant categories	
Zygomatic arch		
simple fracture treatment		
open reduction	D7650	75
closed reduction	D7660	75
compound fracture treatment		
open reduction	D7750	76
closed reduction	D7760	76

PRACTICAL
GUIDE
SERIES

4

Numeric Index to the CDT Code

ADA American Dental Association®
America's leading advocate for oral health

CDT Category		Changes		CDT Category		Changes	
Code	Page	• = Addition ▲ = Revision # = Deletion	Page	Code	Page	• = Addition ▲ = Revision # = Deletion	Page

CDT Category		Changes	
Code	Page	• = Addition ▲ = Revision # = Deletion	Page

I. Diagnostic

Code	Page	Changes	Page
D0120	5		
D0140	5		
D0145	5		
D0150	6		
D0160	6		
D0170	6		
D0171	7		
D0180	7		
D0190	7		
D0191	7		
D0210	7		
D0220	7		
D0230	8		
D0240	8		
D0250	8		
D0251	8		
D0270	8		
D0272	8		
D0273	8		
D0274	8		
D0277	8		
D0310	8		
D0320	8		
D0321	8		
D0322	8		
D0330	8		
D0340	8		
D0350	8		
D0351	9		
D0364	9		
D0365	9		

Code	Page	Changes	Page
D0366	9		
D0367	9		
D0368	9		
D0369	9		
D0370	9		
D0371	9		
D0380	9		
D0381	9		
D0382	9		
D0383	9		
D0384	9		
D0385	10		
D0386	10		
D0391	10		
D0393	10		
D0394	10		
D0395	10		
D0411	10	• Addition	99
D0414	10		
D0415	10		
D0416	10		
D0417	10		
D0418	11		
D0422	11		
D0423	11		
D0425	11		
D0431	11		
D0460	11		
D0470	11		
D0472	12		
D0473	12		
D0474	12		
D0475	12		

CDT Category		Changes		CDT Category		Changes	
Code	Page	● = Addition ▲ = Revision # = Deletion	Page	*Code*	Page	● = Addition ▲ = Revision # = Deletion	Page
D0476	12			D1525	16		
D0477	13			D1550	16		
D0478	13			D1555	16	▲ Revision	101
D0479	13			D1575	17		
D0480	12			D1999	17		
D0481	13						

III. Restorative

CDT Category		Changes	
D0482	13		
D0483	13		
D0484	13		
D0485	13		
D0486	12		
D0502	13		
D0600	11		
D0601	11		
D0602	11		
D0603	11		
D0999	13		

II. Preventive

CDT Category		Changes	
D1110	15		
D1120	15		
D1206	15		
D1208	15		
D1310	15		
D1320	15		
D1330	15		
D1351	16		
D1352	16		
D1353	16		
D1354	16	▲ Revision	101
D1510	16		
D1515	16		
D1520	16		

Restorative table:

CDT Category		Changes	
D2140	20		
D2150	20		
D2160	20		
D2161	20		
D2330	20		
D2331	20		
D2332	20		
D2335	20		
D2390	20		
D2391	20		
D2392	20		
D2393	21		
D2394	21		
D2410	21		
D2420	21		
D2430	21		
D2510	21		
D2520	21		
D2530	21		
D2542	21		
D2543	21		
D2544	21		
D2610	21		
D2620	21		
D2630	21		
D2642	21		

CDT Category		Changes		CDT Category		Changes	
Code	Page	● = Addition ▲ = Revision # = Deletion	Page	*Code*	Page	● = Addition ▲ = Revision # = Deletion	Page
D2643	22			D2932	23		
D2644	22			D2933	24		
D2650	22			D2934	24		
D2651	22			D2940	24		
D2652	22			D2941	24		
D2662	22			D2949	24		
D2663	22			D2950	24		
D2664	22			D2951	24		
D2710	22			D2952	24		
D2712	22			D2953	24		
D2720	22			D2954	24		
D2721	22			D2955	25		
D2722	22			D2957	25		
D2740	22	▲ Revision	103	D2960	25		
D2750	22			D2961	25		
D2751	22			D2962	25		
D2752	22			D2971	25		
D2780	22			D2975	25		
D2781	22			D2980	25		
D2782	23			D2981	25		
D2783	23			D2982	25		
D2790	23			D2983	25		
D2791	23			D2990	23		
D2792	23			D2999	25		
D2794	23						
D2799	23						

IV. Endodontics

CDT Category		Changes		CDT Category		Changes	
D2910	23			D3110	27		
D2915	23			D3120	27		
D2920	23			D3220	27		
D2921	23			D3221	27		
D2929	23			D3222	28		
D2930	23			D3230	28		
D2931	23			D3240	28		

CDT Category		Changes	
Code	Page	● = Addition ▲ = Revision # = Deletion	Page
D3310	28		
D3320	28	▲ Revision	105
D3330	29	▲ Revision	105
D3331	29		
D3332	29		
D3333	29		
D3346	29		
D3347	29	▲ Revision	105
D3348	29		
D3351	29		
D3352	29		
D3353	30		
D3355	30		
D3356	30		
D3357	30		
D3410	30		
D3421	30	▲ Revision	105
D3425	30		
D3426	31	▲ Revision	105
D3427	31		
D3428	31		
D3429	31		
D3430	31		
D3431	31		
D3432	31		
D3450	31		
D3460	31		
D3470	31		
D3910	32		
D3920	32		
D3950	32		
D3999	32		

CDT Category		Changes	
Code	Page	● = Addition ▲ = Revision # = Deletion	Page
V. Periodontics			
D4210	33		
D4211	33		
D4212	34		
D4230	34	▲ Revision	107
D4231	34	▲ Revision	107
D4240	34		
D4241	34		
D4245	35		
D4249	35		
D4260	35		
D4261	35		
D4263	36		
D4264	36		
D4265	36		
D4266	36		
D4267	37		
D4268	37		
D4270	37		
D4273	37		
D4274	38		
D4275	37		
D4276	38		
D4277	38		
D4278	38		
D4283	37		
D4285	38		
D4320	38		
D4321	38		
D4341	39		
D4342	39		

CDT Category		Changes		CDT Category		Changes	
Code	Page	● = Addition ▲ = Revision # = Deletion	Page	Code	Page	● = Addition ▲ = Revision # = Deletion	Page
D4346	39			D5610		# Deletion	109
D4355	39	▲ Revision	107	D5620		# Deletion	109
D4381	40			D5611	43	● Addition	109
D4910	40			D5612	43	● Addition	109
D4920	40			D5621	43	● Addition	109
D4921	40			D5622	43	● Addition	109
D4999	40			D5630	43		

VI. Prosthodontics (removable)

CDT Category		Changes		CDT Category		Changes	
Code	Page	Changes	Page	Code	Page	Changes	Page
				D5640	43		
				D5650	43		
				D5660	43		
D5110	41			D5670	43		
D5120	41			D5671	43		
D5130	41			D5710	43		
D5140	41			D5711	43		
D5211	41			D5720	43		
D5212	41			D5721	43		
D5213	41			D5730	44		
D5214	41			D5731	44		
D5221	41			D5740	44		
D5222	42			D5741	44		
D5223	42			D5750	44		
D5224	42			D5751	44		
D5225	42			D5760	44		
D5226	42			D5761	44		
D5281	42			D5810	44		
D5410	42			D5811	44		
D5411	42			D5820	44		
D5421	42			D5821	44		
D5422	42			D5850	45		
D5510		# Deletion	109	D5851	45		
D5511	43	● Addition	109	D5862	45		
D5512	43	● Addition	109	D5863	45		
D5520	43						

CDT Category		Changes		CDT Category		Changes	
Code	Page	• = Addition ▲ = Revision # = Deletion	Page	Code	Page	• = Addition ▲ = Revision # = Deletion	Page
D5864	45			D5953	54		
D5865	45			D5954	53		
D5866	45			D5955	53		
D5867	45			D5958	53		
D5875	45			D5959	53		
D5899	45			D5960	54		

VII. Maxillofacial Prosthetics

CDT Category		Changes		CDT Category		Changes	
D5982	55						
D5983	56						
D5984	54						
D5911	48			D5985	53		
D5912	48			D5986	56		
D5913	50			D5987	47		
D5914	47			D5988	55		
D5915	52			D5991	56		
D5916	52			D5992	47		
D5919	48			D5993	47		
D5922	50			D5994	56		
D5923	52			D5999	56		

VIII. Implant Services

CDT Category		Changes	
D5924	47		
D5925	48		
D5926	50	D6010	57
D5927	47	D6011	57
D5928	52	D6012	57
D5929	48	D6013	57
D5931	51	D6040	57
D5932	50	D6050	58
D5933	51	D6051	59
D5934	49	D6052	59
D5935	49	D6055	59
D5936	51	D6056	59
D5937	55	D6057	59
D5951	49	D6058	60
D5952	54	D6059	60

CDT Category		Changes	
Code	Page	● = Addition ▲ = Revision # = Deletion	Page
D6060	60		
D6061	60		
D6062	60		
D6063	60		
D6064	61		
D6065	61		
D6066	61		
D6067	61		
D6068	61		
D6069	61		
D6070	61		
D6071	62		
D6072	62		
D6073	62		
D6074	62		
D6075	62		
D6076	62		
D6077	62		
D6080	63		
D6081	63	▲ Revision	113
D6085	63		
D6090	63		
D6091	63		
D6092	63		
D6093	63		
D6094	61		
D6095	63		
D6096	63	● Addition	113
D6100	58		
D6101	58		
D6102	58		
D6103	58		
D6104	58		

CDT Category		Changes	
Code	Page	● = Addition ▲ = Revision # = Deletion	Page
D6110	59		
D6111	59		
D6112	59		
D6113	59		
D6114	59		
D6115	59		
D6116	59		
D6117	60		
D6118	60	● Addition	113
D6119	60	● Addition	113
D6190	57		
D6194	62		
D6199	64		

IX. Prosthodontics, Fixed

D6205	65		
D6210	65		
D6211	65		
D6212	65		
D6214	65		
D6240	65		
D6241	65		
D6242	65		
D6245	65		
D6250	65		
D6251	65		
D6252	65		
D6253	65		
D6545	66		
D6548	66		
D6549	66		
D6600	66		
D6601	66		

CDT Category		Changes		CDT Category		Changes	
Code	Page	• = Addition ▲ = Revision # = Deletion	Page	Code	Page	• = Addition ▲ = Revision # = Deletion	Page
D6602	66			D6920	68		
D6603	66			D6930	68		
D6604	66			D6940	68		
D6605	66			D6950	68		
D6606	66			D6980	68		
D6607	66			D6985	68		
D6608	66			D6999	68		
D6609	66						

X. Oral and Maxillofacial Surgery

CDT Category		Changes		CDT Category		Changes	
D6610	66			D7111	69	▲ Revision	117
D6611	66			D7140	69		
D6612	66			D7210	69		
D6613	66			D7220	69		
D6614	66			D7230	69		
D6615	66			D7240	69		
D6624	66			D7241	69		
D6634	66			D7250	70		
D6710	67			D7251	70		
D6720	67			D7260	70		
D6721	67			D7261	70		
D6722	67			D7270	70		
D6740	67			D7272	70		
D6750	67			D7280	70		
D6751	67			D7282	70		
D6752	67			D7283	70		
D6780	67			D7285	71		
D6781	67			D7286	71		
D6782	67			D7287	71		
D6783	67			D7288	71		
D6790	67			D7290	71		
D6791	67			D7291	71		
D6792	67			D7292	71		
D6793	67						
D6794	67						

CDT Category		Changes		CDT Category		Changes	
Code	Page	● = Addition ▲ = Revision # = Deletion	Page	Code	Page	● = Addition ▲ = Revision # = Deletion	Page
D7293	71			D7530	75		
D7294	71			D7540	75		
D7295	71			D7550	75		
D7296	72	● Addition	117	D7560	75		
D7297	72	● Addition	117	D7610	75		
D7310	72			D7620	75		
D7311	72			D7630	75		
D7320	72			D7640	75		
D7321	72			D7650	75		
D7340	73			D7660	75		
D7350	73			D7670	75		
D7410	73			D7671	76		
D7411	73			D7680	76		
D7412	73			D7710	76		
D7413	73			D7720	76		
D7414	73			D7730	76		
D7415	73			D7740	76		
D7440	73			D7750	76		
D7441	73			D7760	76		
D7450	73			D7770	76		
D7451	74			D7771	76		
D7460	74			D7780	76		
D7461	74			D7810	77		
D7465	73			D7820	77		
D7471	74			D7830	77		
D7472	74			D7840	77		
D7473	74			D7850	77		
D7485	74			D7852	77		
D7490	74			D7854	77		
D7510	74			D7856	77		
D7511	74			D7858	77		
D7520	74			D7860	77		
D7521	74			D7865	77		

CDT Category		Changes	
Code	Page	● = Addition ▲ = Revision # = Deletion	Page
D7870	78		
D7871	78		
D7872	78		
D7873	78		
D7874	78		
D7875	78		
D7876	78		
D7877	78		
D7880	78		
D7881	78		
D7899	78		
D7910	79		
D7911	79		
D7912	79		
D7920	79		
D7921	79		
D7940	79		
D7941	79		
D7943	79		
D7944	79		
D7945	79		
D7946	80		
D7947	80		
D7948	80		
D7949	80		
D7950	80		
D7951	80		
D7952	80		
D7953	80		
D7955	81		
D7960	81		
D7961	81		
D7963	81		

CDT Category		Changes	
Code	Page	● = Addition ▲ = Revision # = Deletion	Page
D7970	81		
D7971	81		
D7972	81		
D7979	81	● Addition	117
D7980	81	▲ Revision	117
D7981	82		
D7982	82		
D7983	82		
D7990	82		
D7991	82		
D7995	82		
D7996	82		
D7997	82		
D7998	82		
D7999	82		

XI. Orthodontics

CDT Category		Changes	
Code	Page	● = Addition ▲ = Revision # = Deletion	Page
D8010	83		
D8020	83		
D8030	83		
D8040	83		
D8050	84		
D8060	84		
D8070	84		
D8080	84		
D8090	84		
D8210	85		
D8220	85		
D8660	85		
D8670	85		
D8680	85		
D8681	85		
D8690	85		

CDT Category		Changes		CDT Category		Changes	
Code	Page	• = Addition ▲ = Revision # = Deletion	Page	Code	Page	• = Addition ▲ = Revision # = Deletion	Page
D8691	85			D9911	90		
D8692	85			D9920	90		
D8693	85			D9930	90		
D8694	85			D9932	91		
D8695	85	• Addition	119	D9933	91		
D8999	86			D9934	91		

XII. Adjunctive General Services

CDT Category		Changes		CDT Category		Changes	
Code	Page	• = Addition ▲ = Revision # = Deletion	Page	Code	Page	• = Addition ▲ = Revision # = Deletion	Page
D9110	87			D9935	91		
D9120	87			D9940	91		
D9210	87			D9941	91		
D9211	87			D9942	91		
D9212	87			D9943	91		
D9215	87			D9950	91		
D9219	87			D9951	91		
D9222	87	• Addition	121	D9952	92		
D9223	88	▲ Revision	122	D9970	92		
D9230	88			D9971	92		
D9239	88	• Addition	121	D9972	92		
D9243	88	▲ Revision	122	D9973	92		
D9248	88			D9974	92		
D9310	89			D9975	92		
D9311	89			D9985	92		
D9410	89			D9986	92		
D9420	89			D9987	92		
D9430	89			D9991	92		
D9440	89			D9992	93		
D9450	89			D9993	93		
D9610	90			D9994	93		
D9612	90			D9995	93	• Addition	121
D9630	90			D9996	93	• Addition	121
D9910	90			D9999	93		